PILATES
FOR SEXUAL ENHANCEMENT

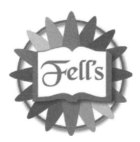

Frederick Fell Publishers, Inc.
2131 Hollywood Blvd., Suite 305
Hollywood, FL 33020
www.Fellpub.com

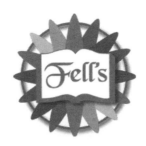

Frederick Fell Publishers, Inc.
2131 Hollywood Blvd., Suite 305
Hollywood, FL 33020
www.Fellpub.com

Please consult a health care professional before starting a new Pilates and/or fitness program, especially if you have current health issues, serious injury or illness. Not all exercises are suitable for everyone. This Pilates program or any fitness program can result in injury. Reduce injury by modifying the exercises, working without force or strain and go at your own pace and skill level. We recommend reading the whole book before performing the exercises.

In addition please consult a health care professional before starting any new diet consisting of new foods, spices and herbs. Our book offers suggestions for foods, spices and herbs. If you question any of the diet suggestions for yourself please consult a doctor before ingesting or using on the body.

For more information about special discounts for bulk purchases. Please contact Fredrick Fell Special Sales at Business@fellpublishers.com.

Cover Design By : Social Agency - www.socialagencyinc.com
Interior Design By : Social Agency - www.socialagencyinc.com

Manufactured in the United States of America.

Library of Congress Cataloging-in-Publication Data

Hershman, Dana, 1969-
  Pilates for sexual enhancement, 8 weeks to a new you and a great sex life / Dana Hershman and Belinda McDonald.
       p. cm.
   Includes index.
   ISBN 978-0-88391-261-4
1. Pilates method. I. McDonald, Belinda, 1973- II. Title.
   RA781.4.H475 2012
   613.7192--dc23

PILATES

FOR SEXUAL ENHANCEMENT

WELL EXPLAINED EXCERCISES AND GUIDED IMAGERY FOR EACH EXCERCISE AND THEIR PROGRESSIONS

CLEAR EXPLANATION OF THE VALUE OF THE EXCERCISES FROM A MEDICAL PERSPECTIVE

A SIMPLE GUIDE TO BUILD FLEXIBILITY AND STRENGTH FOR AN IMPROVED SEXUAL EXPERIENCE

8 WEEKS TO A **NEW YOU** AND A GREAT *SEX LIFE!*

Start Now!

"Dana, thank you for introducing me to Pilates. Pilates has helped my body back in motion after injury."
- Gilad Janklowitz / ESPN-Bodies In Motion

DANA HERSHMAN & BELINDA MCDONALD PT COMT

Dedication

To men and women everywhere, and to all our participants and clients for helping us test our theory.

Acknowledgements

A special thank you to all my clients and friends through the years. Your dedication, commitment to your health, your faith and trust in me as an instructor, confidante and friend keeps me inspired and motivated. Thank you for allowing me to help you in your quest to optimal health and vitality.

To Linda M. Pyle for answering all my writing questions and assuring me to stay focused on the final project, a beautiful successful publication.

To Don Lessne of Frederick Fell who believed in our book and his patience to get the project done right, and to Kim Coffey for being a wonderful and patient editor. Thank you to Kevin Rockwood for his beautiful photography and Karen Belcher for her lovely illustrations and to Scott Bowie for his fabulous photo shop work.

A special thank you to my mentor, Sandy, for always guiding me and being there for me, no matter where my life choices take me.

Dana Hershman

To my husband and best friend, Stephen, thank you for your infinite patience and love.

Belinda McDonald

Table of Contents

"The Pilates is paying off, by the way."

- A happy Alec Baldwin to Meryl Streep in *It's Complicated* after a night of apparently great sex.

Introduction

As a Pilates instructor for over 15 years, I have been to my clients a trainer, friend, drill sergeant, and confidante. Most of my many loyal clients, during the years, have come from all walks of life, doctors, lawyers, CEOs, athletes, dancers, teachers and stay at home moms, to name a few.

Many of them I see more regularly than they see their friends or spouses, and over time my job as a Pilates instructor can turn into therapist and overall confidante. As my relationships with my clients grew and their practice developed, their body and mind began to change. They grew stronger, more flexible and more confident in the body and its capabilities. As a trusted teacher, friend and confidante I heard many stories about friends, family, and trials and tribulations. But the biggest issue that they revealed to me was regarding their sex lives. Whether good, bad, infrequent, fabulous or painful at times they all said that Pilates changed their sex life for the better. They all concluded that Pilates gave them a better sense of their bodies, more confidence and for many a less painful and more enjoyable sexual experience. Many noticed a change right away, others took a little longer but they all noticed a distinct difference after starting a regular Pilates practice.

So, I approached Belinda McDonald, a physical therapist I have the pleasure of working with, and asked her about issues that she was seeing with sexual dysfunction, pain, etc. and the improvements that were made through physical therapy and Pilates.

We decided to conduct a short, fun study to validate our personal findings. Our study consisted of 8 exercises to be done on a daily basis over an 8 week period. Participants varied from those who had never done Pilates to some seasoned Pilates practitioners. Yet, all of them had never taken the time to notice if doing Pilates had changed their sex life. They were eager to start a daily Pilates practice and find out how great their sex life could be.

It turned out that Pilates made a huge difference in all of our participants' sex lives. They gained more strength, flexibility, confidence, and felt healthier and happier overall. In addition, we heard that their spouses were also happy and were more than willing to make sure that the participants maintained their Pilates practice everyday!

So, here is your chance to make a difference in your life and your sex life. By applying the Pilates principles and exercises we believe you will feel better, look better, and rejuvenate your sex life. If your sex life is great already, then applying these Pilates principles and creating a daily practice can only make it better!

"The mind, when housed within a healthful body, possesses a glorious sense of power."

- JOSEPH PILATES

CHAPTER ONE

How Pilates Enhances Your Sexual Function and Improves Function of the Pelvic Floor Muscles

As we move forward in medical science, the most amazing thing I have seen in 17 years as a practicing Physical Therapist, is how incredible the body is without medicinal intervention. I was introduced to Pilates as a weight-loss program over 9 years ago, and it worked! As I continued to use it and apply the principles to my patients, I realized that it was so much more than a weight loss program. I had always been someone who would do heavy aerobic cardiovascular exercises for weight-loss and fitness. But now I had been doing what appeared to be core strengthening workouts and stretching and I had lost weight. The additional advantage was I felt great too!

Over the past 9 years that I have been practicing Pilates and using the concepts with my patients, I also noticed some patients commenting on how not only did the Pilates help them stay strong and flexible, it helped keep pain at bay. In addition, quite a few patients mentioned that it improved their sex life!

Clinically and very randomly I noticed on myself that the range in my neural system had dramatically improved. I was someone, who on school testing, could only bend and touch her knees, now I could forward flex my spine, and get my palms flat on the ground.

I started analyzing and studying why this had occurred. I looked at the individual exercises where the main description indicated stretching. One example is the Pilates exercise Single Straight Leg Pull. When explained by an instructor and when experienced by the individual, it will feel like there is a stretch along the hamstring. But then I noticed that head position or foot position affected these symptoms. So without moving the hamstring, you were changing the sensation experienced. The only explanation I could find was that it was the neural system that was moving differently. What I noticed is that these Pilates exercises tension and slide the nervous system which increases the neural systems movement. This neural system movement increases muscle and overall health of the body and the nervous system.

Pilates is the one exercise program that manages to incorporate the components of pelvic floor exercises and core strengthening exercises. There is great use of the pelvic floor muscles, while engaging and actively using the deep core structures. Base training in pelvic exercises is to independently activate the pelvic floor muscles. Using the Pilates technique daily you gain deep core contraction and control, while controlling the pelvic floor muscles. A longer lasting effect occurs because of overflow from the muscles that are strong and much more functional because these muscles are used daily. These muscles all fire in a synchronized pattern, and Pilates re-educates that function.

From a purely muscular angle, Pilates is wonderful for loaded eccentric activity in a muscle. Eccentric activity is the active lengthening of a muscle, producing a longer leaner muscle. Physiologically this activity increases the metabolic demands on the muscle, much more than a pure concentric contraction. Concentric contraction is the shortening of a muscle that most people end up doing in the gym, like a bicep curl.

The other component that was interesting in regards to the Pilates technique was the lack of repetitions that were encouraged. There are two points that explain the need for fewer repetitions: one that Pilates re-trains muscle memory (one repetition re-educating a muscle is worth 10 mindless contractions). And two, the movements of Pilates are perfect for tensioning and sliding the nerves against the muscle fibers and fascial fibers, and this increases circulation to the nerves, which will optimize function and memory on the muscle and nerve.

Pilates, the Nervous System, and the Anatomy of the Lumbo Pelvic Region - How Their Function Keeps You Healthy and Pain Free

The nervous system is an organ system containing a network of specialized cells called neurons that coordinate the actions of an animal and transmit signals between different parts of its body. In most animals the nervous system consists of two parts, central and peripheral. The central nervous system of vertebrates (such as humans) contains the brain, spinal cord, and retina. The peripheral nervous system consists of sensory neurons, clusters of neurons called ganglia, and nerves connecting them to each other and to the central nervous system. These regions are all interconnected by means of complex neural pathways. The enteric nervous system, a subsystem of the peripheral nervous system, has the capacity, even when severed from the rest of the nervous system through its primary connection by the vagus nerve, to function independently in controlling the gastrointestinal system.

As you can see, the nervous system is a very complex a system all its own. The nervous system will start producing symptoms when it does not move. These symptoms range from restless legs, body aches and pain, to dysfunction in the pelvic floor. That is why it is important to move the nervous system just like you move your muscles and bones.

Joseph Pilates emphasized Pilates as the gateway to complete health and not just physical fitness. Many of the health benefits of Pilates come from the movement Pilates achieves from the pelvis and nervous system.

There are a large number of anatomic structures within the pelvis. Without these, sex is no longer fun, fulfilling and an amazing experience. The building blocks of the pelvis and its support structures are the bony pelvis itself, the muscles outside the pelvis in the buttocks, pelvic floor muscles, pelvic joints (sacroiliac joint and pubic symphysis) and ligaments.

The Nervous System

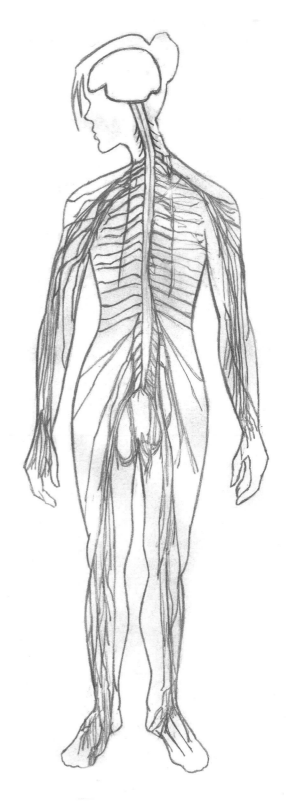

• The pelvic floor is composed of layers of muscles connecting the anterior (front) and posterior (back) portions of the pelvic ring and surrounding the urethra, vagina, and anus. Any layer of the pelvic floor musculature can be the pain generator or the source of dysfunction. Their combined optimal function as a neuromuscular unit is integral to maintaining pelvic floor function. The pelvic floor muscles also contract during orgasm to provide sexual appreciation. But they can be damaged during childbirth, after gynecologic or urologic instrumentation, and even after repetitive minor trauma from activities such as dance and gymnastics. In men, we have seen serious life-altering injuries to the pelvic floor, through compression. Cyclists can develop injury to the pudendal nerve and to the small intrinsic muscles in the pelvic floor.

• The superficial pelvic floor or urogenital diaphragm includes the bulbocavernosus, ischiocavernosus and the transverse perinei.

• The deep pelvic floor or levator ani includes the puborectalis, pubococcygeus, iliococcygeus and the coccygeus.

• The piriformis and obturator internus muscles are often considered associated muscles. The deep transversus abdominus, lumbar multifidi, and diaphragm are synergistic or assisting muscles. The pelvic floor works dynamically in conjunction with these other muscles to maintain core stability. The pelvic floor is considered the "floor of the core".

• Innervation of the pelvic floor in the posterior or back portion is by direct branches from the S2-4 nerve roots, whereas the anterior or front pelvis is innervated by the pudendal nerve and its three branches, the dorsal nerve to the clitoris, the perineal branch and the inferior hemorrhoidal nerve.

Pilates integrates core strengthening and pelvic floor muscle control by reducing the number of repetitions and by coordinating the sequencing of muscle firing. Due to this there is improved control of contraction and release of the pelvic floor structures (eccentric contraction). This control enhances sexual function especially in the individual that experiences pain during intercourse.

Our study

In order to support what our clients felt was occurring, Dana and I thought it would be interesting and fun to do a really easy study with some patients in my physical therapy clinic and some clients of Dana's who all actively enjoyed Pilates. The participants were volunteers, and covered a cross section of the population. Our survey was simple, with a 1-6 rating of their problems and some common issues. The participants rated the issues weekly and kept a daily log of their exercises. We never limited other activities. The study was an addition to their weekly fitness routine. The exercises were carefully selected to enhance the flow of the pelvic movement. The chosen exercises are those that improve the movement of the lower back, and the movement of the neural structures from the root all the way to the terminal endings of the nerve. Many of the participants suffered with back injuries and other orthopedic problems. Many participants were not included in the findings because we saw greater response in getting a drop in pain and improved health. Their sexual function showed some progress however not as significant as those that started with no pain. The clients that started the program with little or no pain are the participants that we listed below who showed the largest change in sexual function.

Results from the survey:

A sample of our questions, which we felt Pilates would really address, is listed below:

1.   Do you do less recreational activities now than you did 5 years ago?
2.   Have you noticed a loss in flexibility over the last 5 years?
3.   Do you have any back pain?
4.   Have you stopped any daily activities because of weakness or pain?
5.   How often do you have sex?
6.   How often would you like to have sex?
7.   Do you have pain with sex?

After the eight weeks we asked people to rate these changes from 1 (no change) to 10 (significant change).

1.   Recreational activity and strength for daily activities: participants rated the changes at 4.5/10.
2.   Flexibility: participants rated the changes 4.5 /10.
3.   Back Pain: participants rated the changes 4.75/10.
4.   Libido: participants rated the changes at 4.5/10.

One aspect, that even in a survey is hard to measure, is the subjective changes. Most participants, even if they could not specify exactly in which way, indicated things had improved. All stated there had been numerous changes. These changes occurred both physically and psychologically with an improved sense of overall well-being. Pilates is known for the toning effect on the legs, and the strengthening of the core muscles. The benefits of the exercises that are often not taken into account are those on the nervous system and on the pelvic region.

Muscle Diagram (Side View) Pelvis, Lumbar, Spine

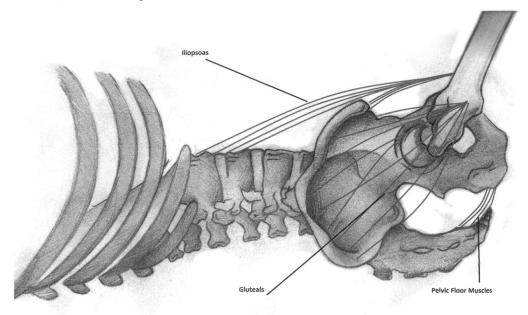

Iliopsoas

Gluteals

Pelvic Floor Muscles

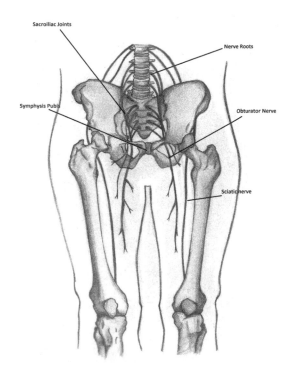

Sacroiliac Joints

Nerve Roots

Symphysis Pubis

Obturator Nerve

Sciatic nerve

Nerve Diagram & Pelvis (Anterior View)

Sexual function is affected by general good health, and the more you can do to improve your health by taking good care of yourself, exercising regularly and eating right the better your sex life can be. Exercise is not only a well documented means of maintaining muscle and losing fat, recent studies propose that it can also revitalize your sex life.

In a February 1999 issue of the *Journal of the American Medical Association*, scientists found that sexual dysfunction is more likely among those with poor physical and emotional health, and plays a major role with negative experiences in sexual relationships and with overall well-being.

Doctors at the New England Research Institute found that regular, vigorous exercise can be effective at lowering impotence risk. The researchers studied more than 600 middle-aged men who hadn't reported any problems with impotence. After eight years, the men who exercised regularly were less likely to have problems.

On the opposite coast, a University of California, San Diego study of 78 healthy but sedentary middle-aged men documented changes when the men were assigned to exercise three to four times a week for one-hour sessions.

Overall, the former couch potatoes reported more reliable sexual functioning, more frequent sexual activity and orgasms, and greater satisfaction.

Yet another study, conducted at the Harvard School of Public Health, revealed that men who exercised vigorously for 20 to 30 minutes were about half as likely to have erection problems as inactive men. The scientists in this study also discovered that as a man gained weight, he became more susceptible to experiencing erectile dysfunction (E.D.).

Women's sex lives can also benefit from regular exercise. Researchers at the University of Texas at Austin studied 35 women, ages 18 to 34. On two separate occasions the women first watched a short travel film, followed by an abbreviated X-rated film. To begin with, the subjects cycled vigorously for 20 minutes. The second time they didn't. Researchers calculated their sexual response using a device that measures blood flow in genital tissue, and discovered that the women's vaginal responses were 169 percent greater after exercising.

In addition, researchers at the University of Cincinnati studied the effect of exercise on reported physical sexual satisfaction of university students. In brief here is what the research had to say:

Research studies that have examined the relationship between exercise and physical sexual satisfaction have all concluded that exercise increases physical sexual satisfaction levels (White, 1990). White found that the men who exercised regularly experienced enhanced sexual encounters including frequency of intimate activities, increased percentages of pleasing orgasms, and sufficient functioning during sex. A recent longitudinal study has found a positive correlation between exercise and sexual satisfaction in women experiencing menopause (Gerber, Johnson, Bunn, & O'Brien, 2005). In addition, women who reported a decrease in frequency of exercise throughout the five year period (of the study) also had a decrease in sexual satisfaction scores. Results of a study on females who began an exercise program revealed an increase in vaginal pulse amplitude and vaginal blood volume in both sexual functioning and sexually impaired women, suggesting that an increase in sympathetic nervous system arousal may produce the outcome of physiological responses in women (Meston & Gorzalka, 1996). Exercise intensifies the sympathetic nervous system thus possibly enhancing physical sexual satisfaction. In a study conducted with cardiac male individuals, researchers concluded that the benefits of exercise training were correlated to improvements in sexual activity (Belardinelli, Lacalaprice, Faccenda, Purcaro, & Perna, in press). Research involving active, older adults similarly found a correlation between physical sexual satisfaction and degree of fitness (Bortz & Wallace, 1999).

Physical Fitness and Improved Sex Life

Pilates is one of the greatest physical fitness programs of our time. As you have read, our study along with numerous other studies on physical fitness clearly concludes that exercise improves one's sex life.

Participating in a regular Pilates program can do many things for your body. Some of the benefits include building strength, flexibility, increased stamina, greater balance, a greater sense of self-confidence, increased body awareness and overall health and vitality. Pilates and participating in a regular fitness program will increase your sexual potency and make sex a lot more fun.

You know that exercise is important to your health, and you read in the earlier chapter that studies, including our study, have found a direct correlation between physical activity, lack of potency and sexual enhancement. Here is an additional list of ways that Pilates will help your fitness level and get the most out of your sex life.

Cardio Endurance

For enthusiastic sex, you'll need to build cardio endurance. It makes your heart strong and keeps your body going. Work on adding 3 or 4 days of cardio exercise like running, walking, swimming or any other activity you enjoy. Adding cardio before your Pilates program will help you boost calorie burning too and help you burn excess fat. In addition, adding cardio to your Pilates routine will get the endorphins going and boost your libido even more.

Muscular Endurance

Sex also requires you to hold unusual positions occasionally for short periods of time, so conditioning your body can be a plus for longer lasting sex. Your Pilates programs will help you build the endurance and flexibility you need for those out of the ordinary postures you may have never tried before.

Strength

Pilates is a basic strength training program that will help you build strength over time. You can challenge your muscles with consistent workouts, and weight bearing exercises like kneeling side work or plank exercises. Remember with Pilates you won't be building the large bulky muscles often associated with great strength. You will build long lean flexible muscles that are strong, balanced and sexy.

Flexibility

Being limber can enhance anyone's sex life by making it a bit easier to get into your favorite positions with a minimum amount of effort. Pilates not only builds amazing strength but also amazing flexibility. In addition to feeling and looking stronger and more toned, you will move with a new found grace and agility. When the body is more flexible you will not feel as stiff and constrained in your body. You will find that you move with less effort and feel lighter and more in tune with your body. Remember to add some Pilates stretches to your cardio or strength training program to maintain and increase your flexibility.

Keep in mind that both sex and exercise have been proven to help reduce stress, doing both on a regular basis should help you stay relaxed and happy. As our study and others have told us exercise also helps increase your sexual desire. Exercise, along with a healthy diet and adequate sleep can boost your libido so you're up for anything.

Sex also burns calories. Of course the sex would have to be fairly vigorous to get your heart rate up, but a 130-lb person can burn about seven calories per five minutes of vigorous sex. Keep it up for an hour, and you'll burn off almost 100 calories! Now that is incentive enough to exercise daily, burn more calories and have amazing sex. What else could you ask for?

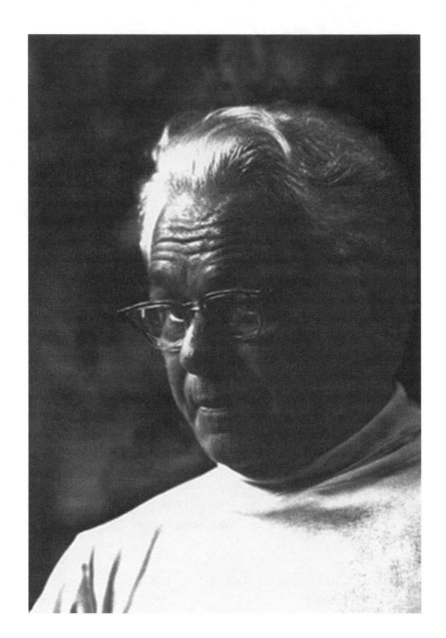

JOSEPH PILATES

"Physical fitness is the first requisite of happiness. Our interpretation of physical fitness is the attainment and maintenance of a uniformly developed body with a sound mind fully capable of naturally, easily, and satisfactorily performing our many and varied daily tasks with spontaneous zest and pleasure."

- JOSEPH PILATES

CHAPTER TWO

Joseph Pilates - À Man Ahead Of His Time

How did the Pilates technique evolve?

I wonder if Joseph Pilates knew how great his technique is for one's sex life? Joseph H. Pilates was born in 1883 in Mönchengladbach, Germany. His father was a prize-winning gymnast of Greek ancestry, and his mother worked as a naturopath. His father's family originally spelled its surname in the Greek manner as "Pilatu" but changed to "Pilates" upon immigration to Germany.

Pilates developed his work from a strong personal experience in fitness. Unhealthy as a child, he studied many kinds of self-improvement systems. He drew from Eastern practices and Zen Buddhism, and was inspired by the ancient Greek ideal of man perfected in development of body, mind and spirit. On his way to developing the Pilates Method, he studied anatomy and developed himself as a body builder, a wrestler, gymnast, boxer, skier and diver.

By the age of 14, he was fit enough to pose for anatomical charts. Pilates came to believe that the "modern" life-style, bad posture, and inefficient breathing lay at the roots of poor health. He ultimately devised a series of exercises and training-techniques and engineered all the equipment, specifications, and tuning required to teach his methods properly.

Pilates was living in England, working as a circus performer and boxer, when he was placed in forced internment in England at the outbreak of WWI. While in the internment camp, he began to develop the floor exercises that evolved into what we now know as the Pilates mat work which is found in this book.

As time went by, Pilates began to work with rehabilitating detainees who were suffering from diseases and injuries. It was invention born of necessity that inspired him to utilize items that were available to him, like bedsprings and beer keg rings, to create resistance exercise equipment for his patients. These were the unlikely beginnings of the equipment we use today, like the reformer and the magic circle.

After WWI, Pilates briefly returned to Germany where his reputation as a physical trainer/healer preceded him. In Germany, he worked briefly for the Hamburg Military Police in self-defense and physical training. In 1925, he was asked to train the German army. Instead, he packed his bags and took a boat to New York City. On the boat to America, he met Clara, a nurse, who would become his wife.

His method, which he and Clara originally called "Contrology," related to encouraging the use of the mind to control muscles. It focuses attention on core postural muscles that help keep the human body balanced and provide support for the spine. In particular, Pilates exercises teach awareness of breath and of alignment of the spine, and strengthen the deep torso and abdominal muscles.

He went on to establish his studio in New York and Clara worked with him as he evolved the Pilates method of exercise, invented the Pilates exercise equipment, and of course, trained students.

Pilates' New York studio put him in close proximity to a number of dance studios, which led to his "discovery" by the dance community. Many dancers and well-known persons of New York depended on Pilates method training for the strength and grace it developed in the practitioner, as well as for its rehabilitative effects. Until exercise science caught up with the Pilates exercise principles in the 1980s, and the surge of interest in Pilates that we have today got underway, it was chiefly dancers and elite athletes who kept his work alive.

Joseph Pilates passed away in 1967. He had maintained a fit physique throughout his life, and many photos show that he was in remarkable physical condition in his older years. He is also said to have had a flamboyant personality. He smoked cigars, liked to party, and wore his exercise briefs wherever he wanted (even on the streets of New York). It is said that he was an intimidating, though deeply committed, instructor. Clara Pilates continued to teach and run the studio for another 10 years after his death.

Pilates Principles

To completely understand the Pilates Method one must understand and apply the 8 principles that make up the core of the Pilates technique. Applying these principles with each exercise makes the movement not just easy to execute but much more effective and energy efficient. The 8 principles must be applied to each exercise with conscious awareness and daily practice.

The eight Pilates Principles are:

Breath
Concentration
Centering
Control
Precision
Fluid motion
Isolation
Focus

1. Breath

"To breathe correctly, you must completely exhale and inhale, always trying very hard to "squeeze" every atom of impure air from your lungs, in much the same manner that you would wring every drop of water from a wet cloth." –Joseph Pilates

Breath is essential not only to fitness but to life. You must breathe through every movement and keep your breath moving in a rhythmic and fluid pattern. Breathing is essential to life and to movement. Breath allows you to move freely without effort and strain. You will notice as you breathe your abdominals will become more active and work more efficiently. Your lungs become stronger and you can gain greater lung capacity. Breath helps cleanse the system of unwanted toxins and bring fresh clean air into the body.

Correct breathing should be performed with the following in mind:

Keep the shoulders, neck and sternum relaxed. Hunching causes neck tension. Keep the breath flowing - do not hold the breath. Breathe in through the nose out through the mouth.

2. Concentration

"The Pilates Method of Body Conditioning is gaining the mastery of your mind over the complete control over your body." - Joseph Pilates

Each movement must be conscious. Ones mind must be clear of distractions and interruptions. Take a few moments before starting your practice to breath deep and bring all your mental and physical energy to yourself. As you move through each exercise watch your body and concentrate on how it is moving. Watch to see that everything is aligned and stable and that you are moving with fluidity and grace.

3. Centering

"Through the Pilates Method of Body Conditioning this unique trinity of a balanced body, mind and spirit can ever be attained. Self confidence follows."
- Joseph Pilates

The abdominal and back muscles area is often described as the core or center. It is the area between the ribs and hips, both anterior (front) and posterior (back) of the torso.

The center is the pivotal point of the body. Execution of each exercise is initiated with awareness of a stable and controlled center. As you progress in your Pilates practice you will see that many exercises take the limbs away from the center of the body. The center must be strong, stable and active to support the limbs moving away from the center. As your core gets stronger you will feel lighter, taller, more balanced and stable. In addition to a centered body, there is balance with mind body and spirit and a feeling of being "centered" and grounded, a feeling of wholeness, self security and personal power.

4. Control

"Ideally, our muscles should obey our will. Reasonably, our will should not be dominated by the reflex of our muscles." - Joseph Pilates

Maintaining control for every movement in Pilates takes concentration, some initial effort and awareness of what the rest of the body is doing at the same time. Repetition, dedication, practice and routine applied daily will improve the degree of control and the perfection of the movement. Not only control is mastered during your practice but a sense of control over the natural functions of the body in everyday life. Body awareness and control are achieved when you create a sense of yourself within your body.

5. Precision

"Correctly executed and mastered to the point of subconscious reaction, these exercises will reflect grace and balance in your routine activities." - Joseph Pilates

The space within which a person moves and performs various physical activities also determines and is determined by precision. Precise movement in your physical activities will also reflect in how you perform daily activities in everyday life. Precision is conscious and unconscious. As you move through your practice you will see, feel and control how precise you can move. Going through the natural movements of everyday life you will achieve a sense internally and externally of how complete, controlled and precise your movements are with little effort. Everyday movements that may have seemed difficult, full of effort and uncomfortable will be performed with precision and fluidity and feel naturally comfortable and effortless in your body.

6. Fluidity

"Pilates, is designed to give you suppleness, natural grace and skill that will be unmistakably reflected in all you do." - Joseph Pilates

Fluid movement, when you exercise, will reflect in fluid movement when you're not exercising. Dynamic, energetic movements replace the static, quick and jerky movements of other techniques. Pilates movements replace speed with fluid controlled consciousness of the body. The execution of the movements should feel smooth with very little effort as is if your body is moving gracefully through water.

The movements of everyday life that may seem hard and unbalanced are replaced with grace, precision and fluidity. Your body will feel and look lighter; you will look taller and leaner. Bulky heavy muscles that lacked strength, form or structure are replaced by long lean flexible muscles that move fluidly and effortlessly.

7. Isolation

"Each muscle may cooperatively and loyally aid in the uniform development of all our muscles." - Joseph Pilates

"True flexibility can be achieved only when all muscles are uniformly developed." - Joseph Pilates

Once there is better control of the weaker muscle groups, more control over the muscles can be obtained and increased isolation of that muscle can be achieved. Enhanced precision of movement is then also possible. Isolation is also about knowing which muscles to stabilize and which to move during a specific exercise. For example in Double Leg Stretch you must learn to isolate and stabilize the trunk or core and move the limbs independently, away from the center of the body.

Apply isolation to everyday movements. The activities you do daily like sitting, or reaching in a cupboard for something does not need the whole body to create the movement though at times it may feel like it. When you know how to isolate and stabilize muscles your everyday actions will seem effortless.

8. Focus

"The Pilates Method of Body Conditioning is gaining the mastery of your mind over the complete control over your body." - Joseph H. Pilates

Focus is understanding and being aware of where you are in the moment, knowing, feeling and moving your body without effort, restrictions or distractions. Focus applies to not just a particular movement but also the focus on the practice as a whole.

Whether your practice is 1 hour long, 15 minutes, consisting of 20 exercises or 8 exercises, focus will help you maintain all the Pilates principles and give you the results you seek.

The Pilates method is about creating improved quality of movement, which in turn creates a greater quality of life.

Creating a daily practice will improve your quality of movement and your quality of life in addition to creating a greater quality of sexual prowess you never imagined.

Who wouldn't want a more fluid, effortless, pleasurable and energetic sexual experience? Using and applying the Pilates principles and our 8 week program will help you achieve that wonderful, physical sexual experience.

Eight simple exercises a day for 8 weeks not just for great sex but for more enjoyment, strength, flexibility and overall health and vitality! Done on a daily basis, alone or as part of your regular fitness program this can be a positive and stimulating change to your physical and sexual fitness and your mind-body connection.

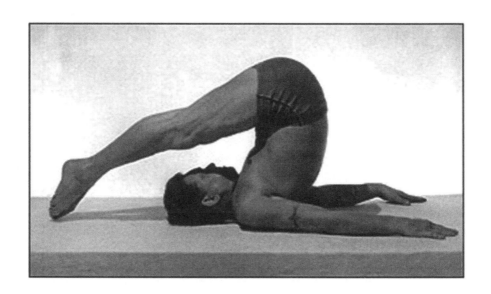

Joseph Pilates doing the Roll Over

"Ideally, our muscles should obey our will. Reasonably, our will should not be dominated by the reflex of our muscles."

- JOSEPH PILATES

CHAPTER THREE

8 Weeks To A New You & A Great Sex Life

Why an 8 week program of 8 exercises?

Over the years, many of my clients have asked for a home program that they can do daily. They want something that can be done using very little space and the most important factor, very little time. Most people want an effective program that can be done in less than a half hour. I have found that when given too many exercises, usually over ten, a person is less likely to maintain a regular routine. Most of the home programs that I develop have less than ten exercises. Over time as a client progresses and builds a habit I add an additional 8 exercises that can be done alone or in addition to the 8 they have already mastered.

Pilates is a very precise and controlled fitness technique. It takes time to develop a strong core and strong mental focus that goes with a daily practice. Every person is different, learns and practices at different rates and abilities. It usually takes about 8 weeks for a beginner to develop the strength, habit and control that is needed for an effective Pilates practice. As you get stronger and move onto Program 2, you can add the 8 exercises to Program 1 that you have mastered or you can just focus on Program 2.

Basically it is your workout. We do recommend staying with each program consistently for 8 weeks before moving onto the next one.

As we put together our study we took into account time, combination of exercises and each program at every level, beginning, intermediate, and advanced. Each exercise we chose moves and stimulates the pelvic floor muscles most effectively. Our participants were from every level of fitness and every level of Pilates. We discovered that an 8 week program would keep participants consistent and give them an adequate amount of exercises where they would notice an improvement in strength, flexibility and sexual prowess.

"Patience and Persistence are vital qualities in the ultimate successful accomplishment of any worthwhile endeavor." - Joseph Pilates

What Does Each Program Do for My Body and Sexual Enhancement?

Each exercise program, 1, 2 and 3 targets every range of motion of the spine: flexion, rotation, extension and lateral flexion. Each individual program consists of 8 exercises designed to work the muscles of the core (abdominals, buttocks and back muscles), the pelvic floor muscles and the nervous system.

Program 1 (Beginning) is a set of 8 basic exercises that will give you a clear understanding of the movement, how it applies to your body and how to execute it properly. After 8 weeks of consistent daily workouts you should notice a change in posture, muscle balance, flexibility and enhanced sexual pleasure. Everyday activities will start to seem easier and be executed with less effort and thought. With more confidence and a better sense of self, your sex life may become more adventurous and stimulating in many ways.

Program 2 (Intermediate) is a set of 8 intermediate Pilates exercises, which are a step up from Program 1. With your new found greater strength and flexibility Program 2 will challenge your body and mind in new ways. You will probably start to notice more development and more strength in the arms and legs. The buttocks will feel more "lifted" and firm. Now that you are getting stronger and gaining more endurance by challenging your body with a more intense program, your endurance in bed may surprise you.

Program 3 (Advanced) is a set of 8 advanced Pilates exercises. Your everyday activities will seem like they were never an issue. A balanced body and sound mind are now a reality and your ability to execute the exercises seems like a piece of cake. Program 3 will challenge your body in ways you may have never used it before. Program 3 will challenge your balance, precision, coordination and strength. Building long, lean, strong flexible muscles is now a reality and Program 3 challenges all that hard work and persistence.

Now that you're ready to tackle this new physical and mental project just a few notes on what to expect with each program:

    - Each exercise includes a step-by-step explanation of how to execute the exercise properly. In addition there is explanation of how to modify the exercise if need be.

    - Each exercise also has a brief explanation of what the exercise does for you on a physical level and how each exercise affects and enhances your sex life.

"Above all, learn how to breathe correctly."

- JOSEPH PILATES

CHAPTER FOUR

Basic Fundamentals & The Essentials Of Body Positioning

Breathing

Breathing is the most important physical principle that you will apply to your movement and to your daily practice. Breath should be practiced as a separate exercise even before you begin your daily routine. Remember breath is vital to every aspect of your body. Clinical practice and scientific evidence suggest that many people develop reduced or incorrect breathing habits over time. This often contributes to lower energy and performance, increased and sustained stress, compromised immune systems and more frequent illnesses.

Most of us change our breath under different circumstances. Sometimes we limit our breath and reduce breath function, misplace breathing patterns and change breath habits that impact health over time. These habits can become associated with imbalance in our muscles, posture, movements and mind body connections.

Breathing has many major functions:
1. Breathing carries nutrients to all body parts, energizing the whole body.
2. Breathing carries waste for elimination from the body.
3. Breathing increases stamina.
4. Breathing relieves stress.

We all have probably experienced ourselves or have seen people in a fitness class hold their breath at the most crucial time and when it can be most beneficial. Holding the breath during exercise is like building pressure in a teakettle. A result of built up pressure is energy and effort wasted. The effect is a muscle that is not utilized effectively because all the mental and physical focus is on the stress the body is undertaking.

Perform breathing fluidly, in through the nose and out the mouth. Keep the shoulders and neck relaxed and focus on breathing into your back allowing the abdominals to stay hollow and active.

Breathe for the life of your body and mind and for effective, efficient effortless movement.

In Pilates we will be practicing a lateral breath, breathing more into the upper part of the trunk, keeping the belly free of air, so you can engage and hollow out the abdominals. There is a sense of breathing into the back of the body without pushing the ribcage out and lifting the sternum. When I cue in class I refer to "knitting the ribs" together as a sense of closing the ribcage and relaxing the sternum to bring the mid back into neutral and help you "imprint" the spine into the mat.

Here is a simple breathing exercise to help you feel your breath more into the back of the body so you can engage and activate the abdominals more effectively.

Sit tall in a chair with your back against the back of the chair or sit tall against a wall on your Pilates mat. Wrap your hands around each side of your ribcage high up on your waist. Close your eyes and take a deep breath in through the nose. Where does your breath go? Into the belly? Does your ribcage lift and "pop out"? Breathe out and feel the belly draw in towards your spine.

Try again. This time as you breathe in, focus on breathing into your hands and into the chair or wall behind you. Do not let the belly fill with air; instead fill the lungs with air. Keep the ribcage "knit together" as if you are tying a shoe. Remember the breath should be long and fluid. Feel the back expand on the wall or chair behind you.

Exhale and expel all the air from the lungs drawing the abdominals deeper towards the spine with a sense of them lifting up and under the ribs. Do not let the shoulders hunch or the back round.

Stay tall and feel a sense of imprinting your back into the wall behind you. This is your sense of neutral spine, which we will address soon.

Practice this breath over and over to give you a better sense of your breath during your practice. You can practice this breath anytime. I like to do it in the car especially when I am stressed and find that I am just not breathing. It gives me a sense of center and relaxes me. But keep your eyes open and your hands on the steering wheel, not your ribcage.

As a rule, always remember to breathe during your Pilates practice. Without breathing during your exercises your practice will feel like a lot more work.

Imprinting, Neutral Position and Pelvic Clock

Before you just jump onto your mat and start your Pilates workout there are a few important body positions and basic body principles you want to master. Those basic body principles are neutral position, imprinting and what I refer to as Pelvic Clock. Having a sense of your body on the mat, your breath, the 8 Pilates Principles and the basic body positions are the backbone of your Pilates practice.

When cuing I refer to the pelvis like a clock. When your pelvis is in neutral all four points of the pelvis should be balanced like a clock, 12, 3, 6 and 9. This is a simple tool to refer back to when you may not be feeling centered or your body is feeling off balance.

The following exercise will help you find your pelvic clock and walk you through imprinting of the spine as well.

Here is a simple exercise you can do to find your "pelvic clock" and one you can return to at anytime to refresh your muscle memory.

Pelvic Clock Exercise

Lie on your back, knees bent and feet flat. Using the image of a marble, balance the marble in the center of your clock between the naval and the pubic bone. The marble should balance there easily. As we go through the steps of the exercise you will use your imagination and your pelvis to roll the marble from one point to the other. This imagery and movement will allow you to gain awareness of where your pelvis should be when in neutral and give you a sense of when you are off center.

The following step-by-step program will walk you through the movements of the "pelvic clock." You will feel a sense of the naval and abdominals "scooping and hollowing" towards the spine with the marble sinking into the naval, just as you did with the breathing exercise.

I always refer back to the Pelvic Clock exercise if I lose track of my center or am feeling unbalanced during my practice.

Since this exercise can seem rigid and slow at times, I like to do this exercise with my eyes closed. Having my eyes closed allows me to release distractions and just focus on the precision and fluidity of the motion. There is a certain sensuality of movement in the pelvis when it moves fluidly and with grace.
During sex the pelvis should be able to relax, feel fluid and graceful yet powerful and strong. The nerves are alive and energized.

Step by step:

1. Lie on your mat, knees bent hip width apart and feet grounded on the floor.
2. With the imaginary marble balanced between the navel and pubic bone take a deep inhale to prepare.
3. Exhale and roll the marble to your naval (12 o'clock). The pubic bone should lift towards the sky and the middle back flattens onto your mat.
4. Inhale and roll the marble back to the center point, neutral.
5. Exhale; roll the marble to the pubic bone (6 o'clock). Your back will be arched with the low back lifted off the floor. Focus in on the abdominals being active to support your spine.
6. Inhale and roll the marble back to the middle of the clock, neutral. Balance the marble in the center of the clock.
7. Exhale and roll the marble to your left hip (3 o'clock). The right hip will naturally lift off of the floor towards the sky, but not towards your shoulder.
8. Inhale and roll the marble back to neutral, balanced between the navel and the pubic bone.
9. Exhale and roll the marble to the right hip (9 o'clock). The left hip will naturally roll off the floor towards the sky, but not towards your shoulder.

Repeat this exercise many times to get a sense of neutral and a sense of when you're not in neutral. You want the pelvis and the spine to feel balanced and centered.

Another fun exercise is to roll the marble to every number on the clock 12, 1, 2, 3…and so on. Maintaining a natural breathing pattern, roll your hips around in a circular motion as if rolling a bowl around on its edge, and then reverse the direction. You may notice one direction moves easier than the other. After a week or so of doing your daily Pilates routine go back to this exercise and see how much easier and smoothly the pelvis moves.

Pelvic Clock

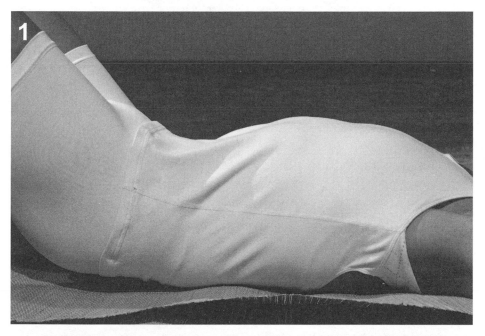

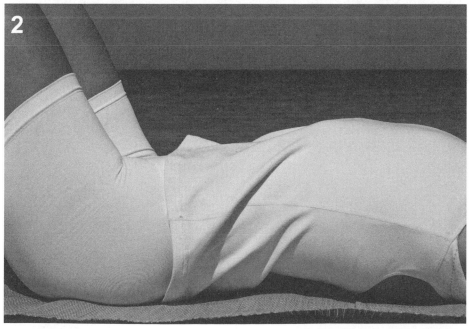

Imprinting and Neutral Position

Imprinting is a tool I use to ground the spine into the mat and prepare your body and trunk for your workout. Start by finding and balancing your pelvic clock.

To begin imprinting I like to use the image of lying in wet sand. Slowly allow your spine to relax into the sand, allowing one vertebrae at a time to soften and relax. Feel the abdominals fall and hollow towards the spine maintaining the pelvic clock position by not tilting the pelvis or rolling.

The shoulders should glide down your back away from your ears connecting to your mid back. You can do this by reaching your arms along your mat towards your feet. You should feel the mid back muscles engage. The ribcage will knit towards each other and the sternum should relax away from the breast bone. Your spine and torso will feel relaxed yet active and ready to workout. The back of the neck should be long and the chin should not lift. If you have tight shoulders or neck muscles add a small towel under your head to help keep your neck and head neutral and your shoulders down.

Most Pilates exercises require neutral position throughout the exercise so it is important to practice and develop muscle memory in the pelvic floor and pelvis area. Plus it feels good to move the pelvis easily and fluidly. Having a mobile, flexible fluid pelvis allows for a more pleasurable sexual experience.

One thing to remember is that not all backs are the same. Depending on your structure, muscle tightness or flexibility your spine may feel and look different than another's when in neutral. Correct neutral also requires the abdominals to be active. As you are breathing your abdominal muscles will start to fire and become active. Take note of what that feels like as you're moving and when you're lying still.

Pilates is designed to get your body to its most functional and capable body and sound mind. Pilates exercises build a strong sturdy body that can perform everyday activities with ease, grace, very little effort and perfection.

Imprinting and Neutral Position

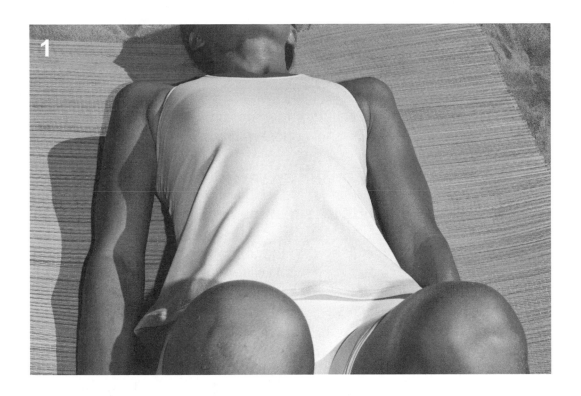

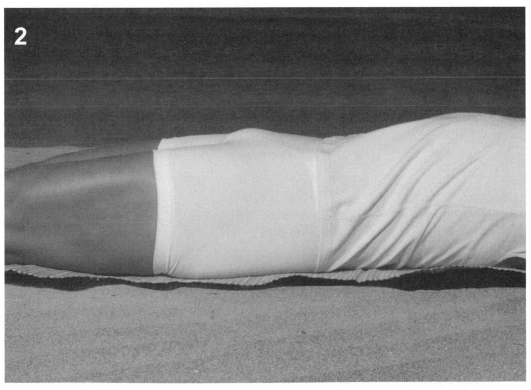

Hammock Technique, a Modification Tool

This is a great technique to use if you have back or neck issues. Or if you are finding that your abdominal muscles are not strong enough yet to fold you into flexion without straining your neck and shoulders. The Hammock Technique is a great tool to use to help your head and shoulders stay more relaxed so you can maintain flexion and perform most Pilates exercises with little effort or muscle strain.

Lie on your mat or a small towel with your head close to the top of the mat, but not completely off of the mat. Hold the corners of the mat or towel keeping your shoulders down and your back and abdominals active. It is important to keep the shoulders down and the back muscles active to aid you as you come up. Remember that your core is made up of muscles in the front and back of your body, and they need to stay active to bring your body into flexion. The arms and neck should not do the work of lifting the head off the mat.

As you activate your abdominals to bring you into flexion the mat will come with you aiding your head and shoulders as you roll forward. The head should feel light and relaxed like lying in a hammock. Try not to pull the mat too hard by using your arms as you lift up. Your abdominals should be doing most of the work and your arms and head just follow.

Use this technique if you're a beginner, or if you are feeling head or neck strain. As you progress and get stronger you can use the Hammock Technique and then drop it half way through the exercise placing the hands behind the head or into the arm position for the particular exercise.

Sometimes, I use the Hammock Technique on myself and with my advanced students when we go "back to basics" to help find a deeper connection with the abdominals. It is easy to get into the habit of using the neck and arms to bring you into flexion. Always remember that the muscles that initiate the spine to move into flexion (forward bending) are the abdominals and back muscles of the trunk.

Now that you have practiced and have an understanding of the basic fundamentals of Pilates it is time to get started on your workouts. Following are the three 8 week programs that we designed to get you into great shape and improve your sex life. Each of the 3 programs contain 8 level appropriate exercises to help you gain strength, flexibility and overall health and vitality. Done on a daily basis, alone or as part of your regular fitness program – this can be a positive and stimulating change to your sexual fitness and mind-body connection.

Remember your ultimate goal is to create a sound mind within a sound body through patience and persistence that exudes amazing grace, self-confidence, and power and enjoys a fulfilling and amazing sex life! Have fun!

Hammock

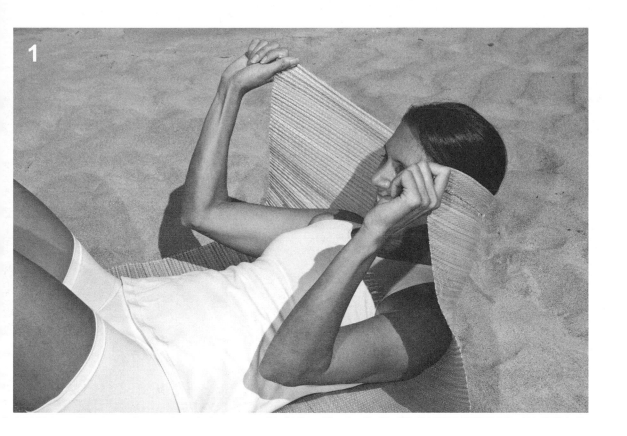

The Sexual Enhancement Workouts

"Patience and persistence are vital qualities in the ultimate successful accomplishment of any worthwhile endeavor."

- JOSEPH PILATES

Program #1
(Beginning)

Program 1 (Beginning)

Program 1 is designed for those who have never practiced Pilates or those who have studied for awhile. This program is a set of 8 basic exercises that will help you gain a sense of your center, your muscles and bones and how important the basic fundamentals are to your Pilates practice. This fundamental program is important to every Pilates practice, beginning to advanced.

Program 1 consists of 8 basic Pilates exercises. Most are modifications of exercises you will do in Programs 2 and 3. All exercises should be executed at your own pace. Read through the entire exercise and modifications and review the photos at least once to create a mental picture of how the exercise is to be executed. Always modify and apply modifications as you need.

Following Program 1 daily for 8 weeks is how you will get the most benefit out of the program and jump start you into forming a life long habit of a daily Pilates routine. Do Program 1 consistently for 8 weeks and you will be on your way to a balanced progressive and effective first program that will help you progress to the next level. Don't forget that the main goal of this program is a new improved better sex life! That should be motivation enough to keep you consistent, focused and progressing beautifully.

The Exercises for Program 1

Bridging
Pendulum- Modified
The Hundred-Modified
Single Leg Stretch
Spine Stretch
Seated Twist
Mermaid
Spinal Wave

Bridging

Spinal Movement: Pull spine articulation.

Step by step:

1. Lie on your back with your knees bent and hip-width apart. The feet are flat on the mat and heels directly under the knees.
2. Inhale to prepare for the movement. Exhale as you slowly articulate the spine off of the mat one vertebra at a time as if you are rolling a marble from the pubic bone to the upper back. Press the pubic bone up to the sky without over extending in the spine. Your heels and toes should be pressed firmly into the mat and legs and buttocks active. Do not let the knees fall open.
3. Inhale, hold the position. Exhale as you slowly roll the spine back down to the mat moving from the upper back through the mid back and back down to the pelvis. Move one vertebra at a time, rolling the imaginary marble back down to the pubic bone. Keep the shoulders down, away from the ears and your arms long along the mat. Make sure you do not over extend the pelvis. Do not roll past your neutral position.
4. Inhale to prepare again, keeping the pelvic clock neutral and spine long. Keep the legs and buttocks active as you roll back up.
5. Repeat the movement 5-8 times.

Pointers for proper execution:

Do move slowly as you focus on peeling your spine off the mat.
Do breath fully through every movement, inhaling and exhaling.
Do focus on keeping your abdominals, legs and buttocks active.
Do keep your focus and keep your head aligned and avoid tilting the head from side to side.

Do not go beyond your range of motion.
Do not let the back arch, shoulders and chin lift.
Do not allow your knees to roll away from neutral alignment with your hips.
Do not tilt back onto your heels. Keep your feet firm on the ground.

Modifications:

Roll only half way up until you feel stronger and more flexible in the spine and core. You can also practice the pelvic clock exercise here until you feel stronger and more capable of lifting and articulating the spine.

How Bridging helps you during sex:

Bridging offers great contraction of the hamstrings and superior control of the pelvic floor muscles (perineum). There is stabilizing in the transverse abdominus while there is lengthening of the abdominals. This is the interaction and rhythm needed for great sex.

How Bridging helps your whole body:

It warms the deep abdominal structures and stimulates the pelvic floor muscles, releasing the pelvic floor while the glutes contract, an action that is helpful in those that suffer with pain during intercourse. The pelvic joints are rotated and compressed to allow better function. In addition, there is gliding of the pelvic and lower back nerves to warm them, without moving the terminal ends, slowly turning up the heat.

Bridging

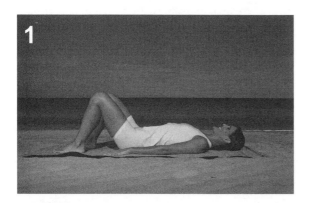

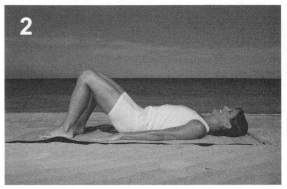

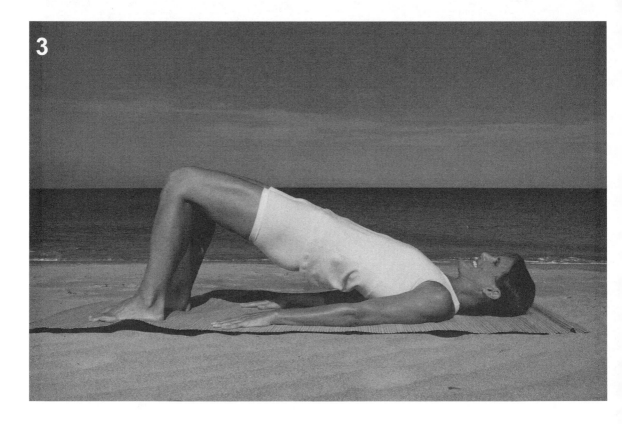

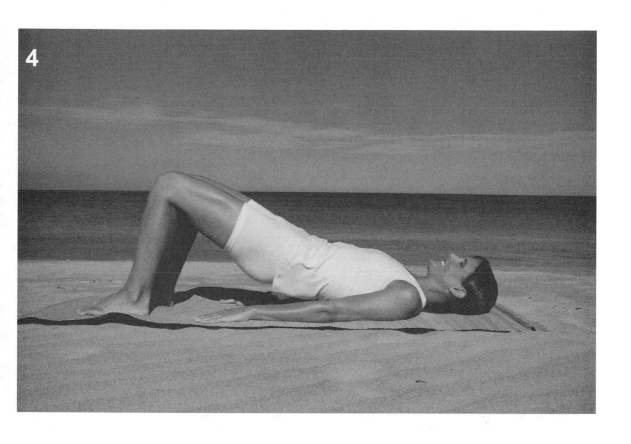

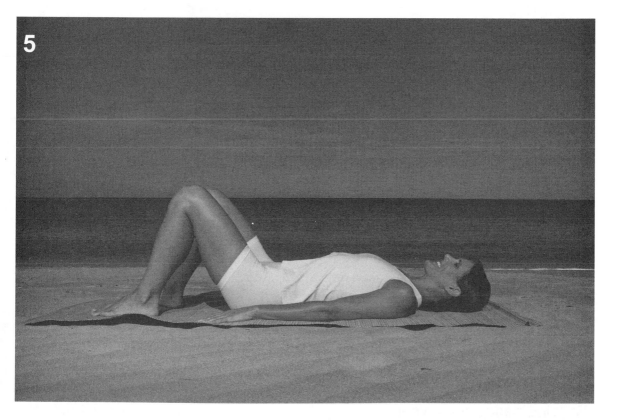

Pendulum - Modified

Spinal Movement: Cervical and thoracic stability, lumbar rotation.

Step by step:

1. Lie on your mat with your arms stretched out in a T position from the shoulders. The spine and pelvis are neutral along the mat. Inhale here to prepare.
2. Exhale as you fold the knees up to a 90 degree angle.
3. Imagine a marble in the belly button, like the pelvic clock exercise. As you inhale, slowly roll the marble to the left hip (or 3 o'clock position). The right hip will lift towards the sky.
4. Exhale and roll the hips back to center initiating from you abdominals not your back.
5. Inhale and roll the marble to the right, 9 o'clock position. The left hip will lift towards the sky.
6. Exhale and roll back to center.

Repeat 6-8 times on each side being careful not to lift the hip towards the shoulder as you twist. Maintain length through the spine at all times.

Pointers for proper execution:

Do keep your head in line with your spine at all times.
Do keep your gaze straight up to the sky.
Do use the back and abdominal muscles to keep the upper trunk still so you can isolate the pelvis.

Do not turn the head side to side.
Do not let the shoulders come off of the floor. Use the trunk muscles to keep the upper trunk still so you can isolate the pelvis.
Do not go so far to one side that you cannot control moving back to center.

Modification:

There is no specific modification for modified pendulum. If you have trouble lifting your feet off of the ground, lift your heels only, keeping the toes on the mat. Follow the same steps and rotate from the hips. You may not get the same range of motion but you will warm up the deep abdominals and the low back, which is one main purpose of modified pendulum.

How Pendulum - Modified helps during sex:

By doing pendulum the perineum and the pelvic floor muscles contract aiding in strong orgasms. The abdominals contract and eccentrically release for greater sexual control.

How Pendulum - Modified helps the whole body:

The large sciatic nerve is tensioned up first, before the side to side movement where it glides through the large piriformes muscle in the hips. There is also great rotation in the large vertebrae of the lumbar spine with segmental control retrained in the abdominals. By rocking back and forth, the large sacroiliac joints are compressed and released loosening up all the nerve roots that supply the pelvic floor muscles. These are the all important muscles to heighten the sexual experience. For the individual that experiences pain during sex, this will help release all the painful structures.

Pendulum - Modified

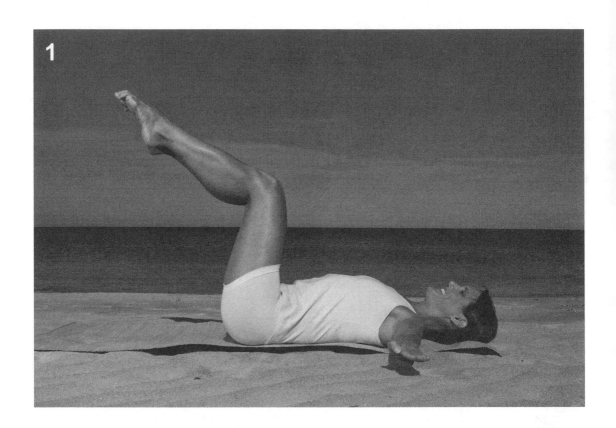

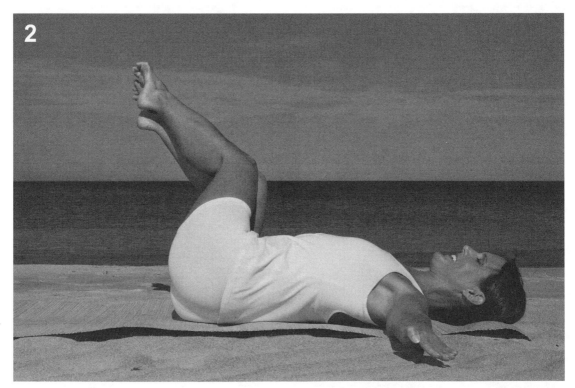

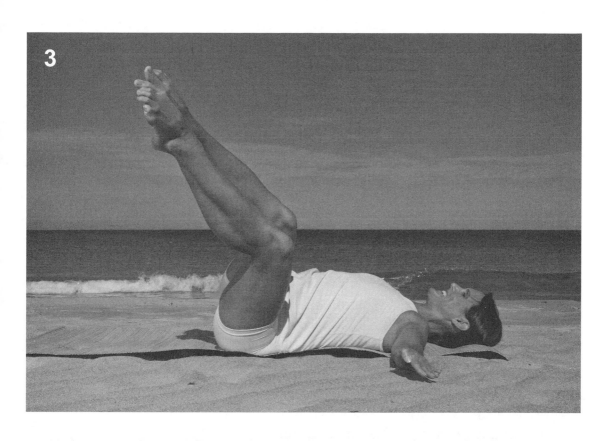

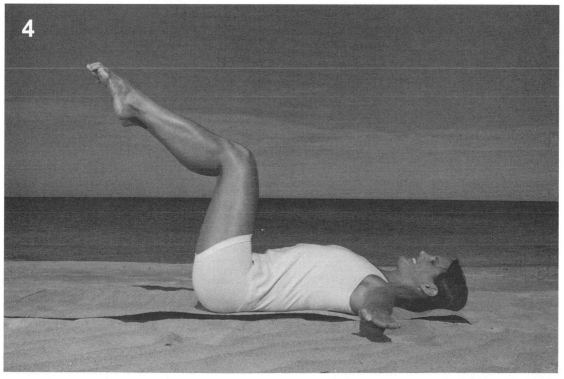

The Hundred - Modified

Spinal Movement: Cervical and upper thoracic flexion, with controlled pelvic positioning.

Step by step:

1. Lie on your back, knees are bent and feet flat. Exhale to activate the abdominals and fold the knees up into a 90 degree angle. Arms are reaching towards the sky shoulder width apart.
2. Inhale to prepare. Exhale and fold the upper trunk into flexion.
3. Pump the arms up and down vigorously as if slapping puddles of water. Inhale deeply for 5 counts and exhale for 5 counts, developing a pumping type breath (diaphragmatic breathing). Five quick inhales and five quick exhales. Your goal is to reach 10 sets of 10 breaths for a total of 100 breaths.
4. After you have reached 100 breaths, inhale deeply as you hold the position. Exhale as you bring the body back down to the mat.

Pointers for proper execution:

Do go slowly at first, gradually building strength and stamina.
Do count your breaths.
Do start with a 2 or 3 count breath and work up to 5.
Do keep your focus on your abdominals.
Do be patient, work up to 100 breaths gradually.

Do not force yourself to do all 100 breaths the first couple of times.
Do not let your shoulders hike to your ears.
Do not compromise on form or breath to get to 100.
Breathe!

Modifications:

Keep your feet on the floor. Keep your head down or use the Hammock Technique to help yourself up. Modify the breathing by taking long breaths in and out. Work up to 5 by starting at 2 or 3 pulses and so on.

How the Hundred - Modified enhances sex:

The Hundred warms up the deepest layer of the abdominals with a strong contraction of the pelvis. This intense warming of the pelvic floor is what we need for great sex.

How the Hundred - Modified helps your entire body:

Creates deep abdominal and core strengthening, and increases the stabilization function in the pelvic floor. The small oscillations warm the entire nervous system, improving blood flow and allowing for great gliding of the nerves against the muscles and joints. The breathing is important – muscles and nerves will not remember movements as easily as they do when they are starved for oxygen and here we immediately create great blood flow and oxygen for the entire body.

Hundred Modified

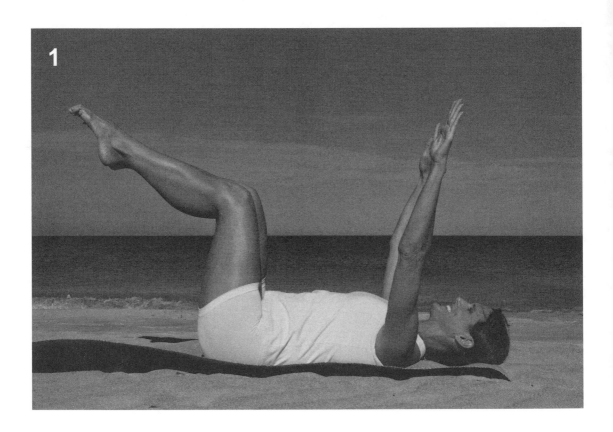

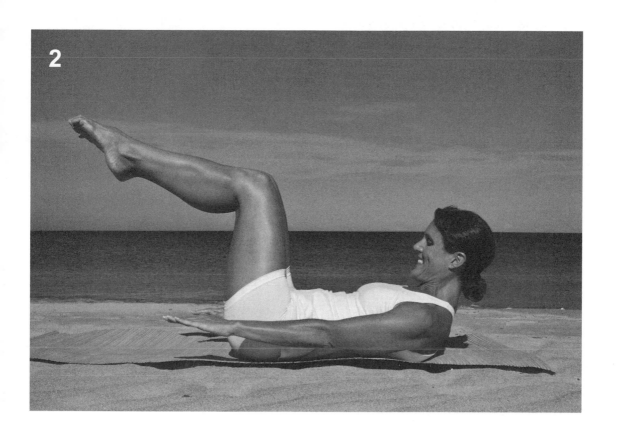

Single Leg Stretch

Spinal Movement: Flexion of cervical and upper thoracic. Lumbar and sacral stability.

Step by step:

1. Lie on your back with your knees bent and feet on the floor. Exhale and fold the legs into a 90 degree angle holding onto the back of the knees.
2. Inhale here as you prepare to move.
3. Exhale. Fold into flexion using your abdominals. Do not pull with the arms or hands.
4. Inhale and hold the position.
5. Exhale. Bring the right knee towards your chest as the left leg reaches long, straight out from the hip. The hips should stay neutral along the mat.
6. Inhale. Draw the left leg back to the start position.
7. Exhale, keeping the left knee bent and hips neutral, reach the right leg out straight from the hip.
8. Inhale and return to your start position.
9. Repeat 5-8 extensions per leg, alternating the breath and the legs from right to left, extending the legs completely as you reach.
10. Finish by pulling both legs into a 90 degree angle and resting on the mat.

Pointers for proper execution:

Do keep your abdominals hollow and scooping towards the spine.
Do keep your spine and hips neutral
Do rest your head if you need to do so, but keep the legs and breath moving.
Do keep your elbows wide to maintain the integrity in your back muscles and to avoid weak arms.

Do not let your extended leg fall below hip level.
Do not let your shoulders hike to your ears.
Do not twist or rotate towards the bent knee; keep your trunk centered.

Modification:

If you feel strain in your neck or back, lower the head back to the mat or use the Hammock Technique. It is best to lift the legs slightly higher with the head down to avoid too much hyperextension of the back. This also keeps the abdominals active. Once you get stronger you can lift the head again and lower the legs slightly. Always maintain the integrity of your spine and abdominals.

How Single Leg Stretch enhances sex:

We all know that we need good hamstring range for an improved sexual experience from foreplay to orgasm. The more flexible you are the better sex will be. Single Leg Stretch builds coordination, flexibility and endurance.

How Single Leg Stretch helps your entire body:

There is incredible gliding of the sciatic nerve roots across the hip as the nerve roots are grounded by a strong contraction of the deep abdominal structures. The foot position allows for great slide of the ends of the nerves against all the muscles in the front of the foot. The benefit for our sex life and pelvic function is how the pelvic floor actively lengthens while there is movement - contraction and eccentric (lengthening) contraction - of the big hip muscles – like the gluteals and hamstrings. For enhancement of sex these muscles have to be able to be strong while working independently. For other areas of life, like bladder control this is a very significant exercise.

Single Leg Stretch

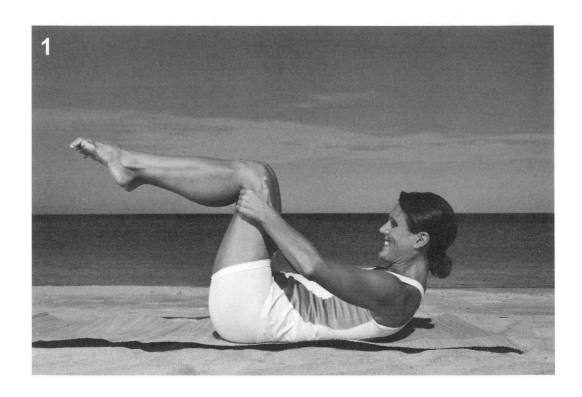

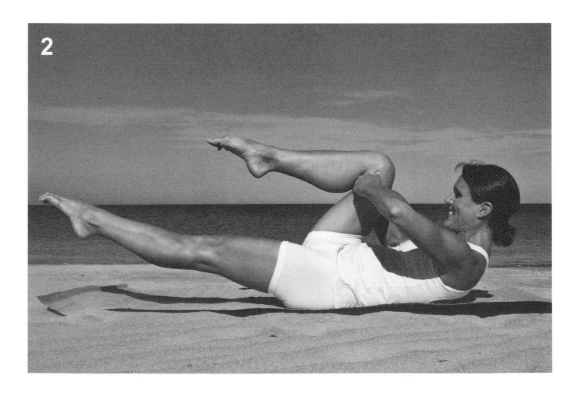

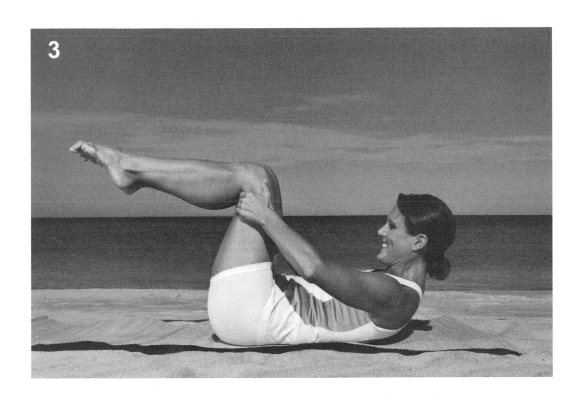

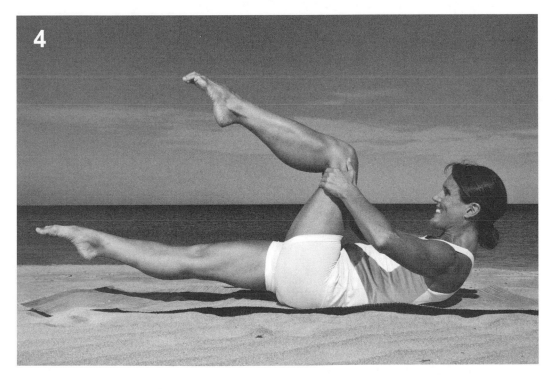

Spine Stretch

Spinal Movement: Forward flexion of the cervical and thoracic spine. Lower lumbar and sacral stability.

Step by step:

1. Start in a seated position with legs outstretched about the width of your mat apart.
2. Inhale as you stretch your arms out in front of you, parallel to the ground, making sure to keep your shoulders back and head neutral as if seated against a wall.
3. Exhaling, peel your spine, head first, away from the imaginary wall behind you, slowly articulating forward from the abdominals into a hollow C-curve position. Make sure the hip bones stay glued to the floor. In other words, don't let your butt come off the mat.
4. Inhale again at your full C curve position.
5. Exhale as you slowly articulate back up to a seated position. Feel your ribs float effortlessly, like a cloud, on top of your hips.
6. Repeat 5-8 times.

Pointers for proper execution:

Do sit up tall and feel yourself grounded into the floor.
Do lead from your abdominals not with your arms.
Do feel the movement initiated from your center.
Do feel your spine and hamstrings stretching.
Breathe!!

Do not slouch.
Do not lead from your arms.
Do not let the knees roll inward.

Modifications:

Sit on a rolled up mat, bolster or pillow to give your hips a lift and bend the knees slightly. This will make it easier to sit up straight and ease tension in your legs.

How Spine Stretch enhances sex:

There is a deep pelvic contraction with a strong pelvic tilt forward. With this pelvis control and overall flexibility sex becomes more powerful and more erotic!

How Spine Stretch helps your entire body:

With the sciatic nerve and its branches placed on full stretch, wonderful gliding occurs in the whole spinal cord, creating healthy blood flow and function. Hamstrings lengthen actively, allowing the big sciatic nerve to glide to full range, and hip flexors lengthen for the deep abdominals to massage the pelvic structures.

Spine Stretch

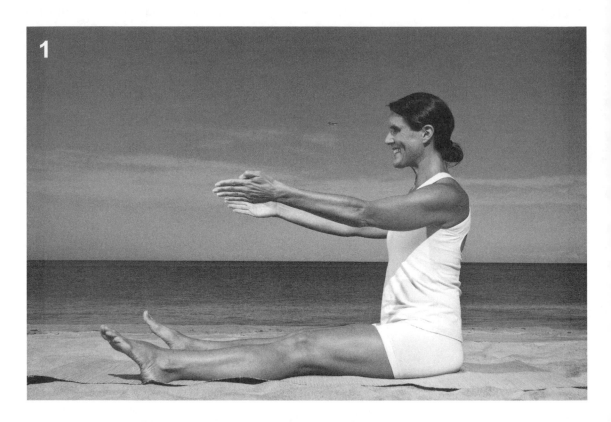

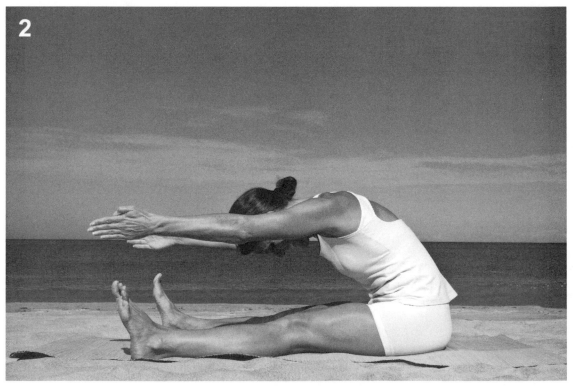

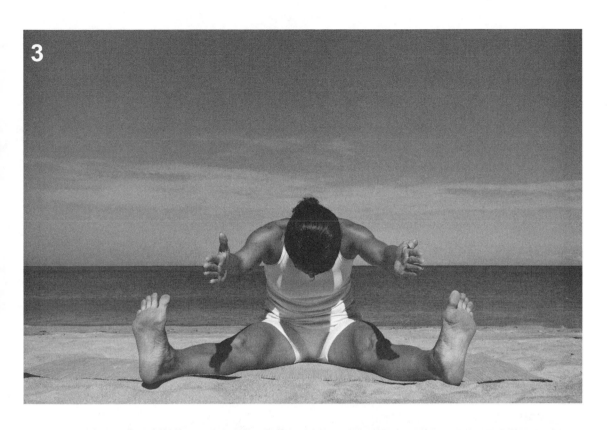

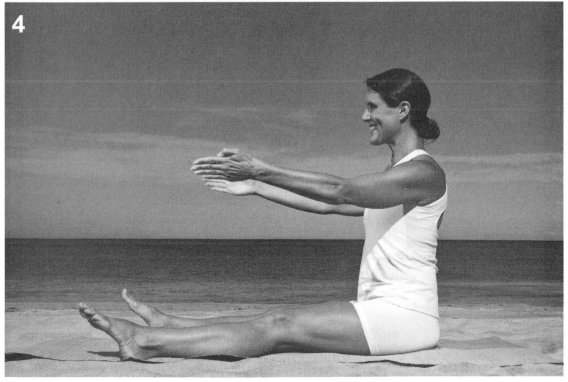

Seated Twist

Spinal Movement: Cervical, thoracic and some lumbar rotation. Lower lumbar and sacral stability.

You can transition right from Spine Stretch into this exercise.

Step by step:

1. Start in a seated position, legs about the width of your mat apart. Extend the arms like a T, as if you are reaching to opposite ends of the room
2. Inhale as you prepare for the movement.
3. Exhale and twist the upper trunk towards the right leg. Keep the arms extending, reaching long away from the body and keep the hips grounded.
4. Inhale and return to the center.
5. Exhale and twist towards the left leg.
6. Inhale and return to center.
7. Alternate right and left 5-8 times per side.

Pointers for proper execution:

Do keep your hips firmly grounded.
Do feel your abdominals wringing out like a wet rag.
Do let your head follow your movement.
Do keep the arms outstretched like a T from the shoulders.

Do not move the hips.
Do not hunch your shoulders.
Do not round your back.
Do not slouch.
Do not let your arms lead or swing out in front of you.

Modifications:

If you cannot sit up straight bend the knees slightly and sit on a rolled up mat or towel. Or cross your legs in front of you. Also, cross the arms in front of you and away from the body slightly. You can also hold onto a small ball or towel with your arms stretched out in front of you.

How Seated Twist enhances sex:

Holding the pelvis in a strong flexed position the hamstrings stretch, holding a strong contraction. There is alternating control of the oblique muscles. Seated Twist is one of the few exercises that gains a strong contraction of the back extensor muscles without which sex would be mediocre at best.

How Seated Twist helps the whole body:

Seated Twist helps strengthen and stretch the oblique muscles and stabilize the pelvic floor muscles. Twisting motions help whittle the waist, lengthen the spine and flatten the belly.

Seated Twist

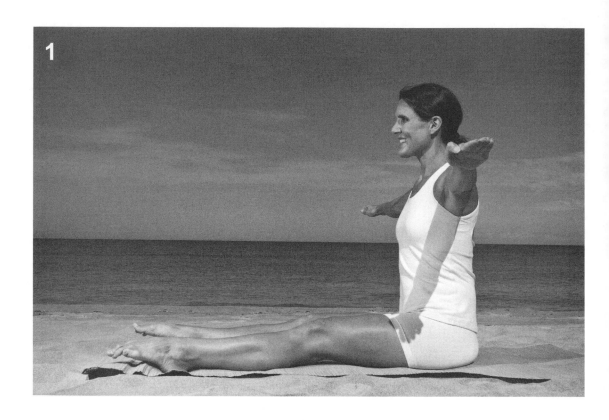

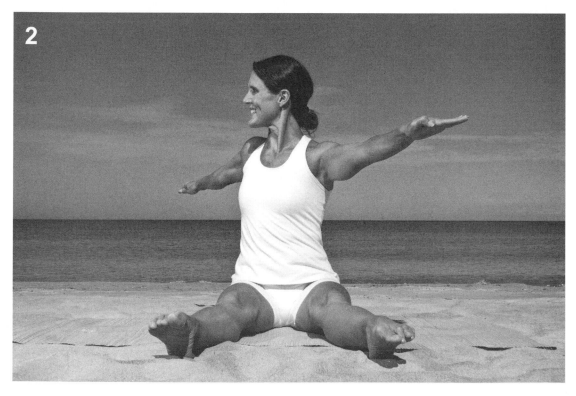

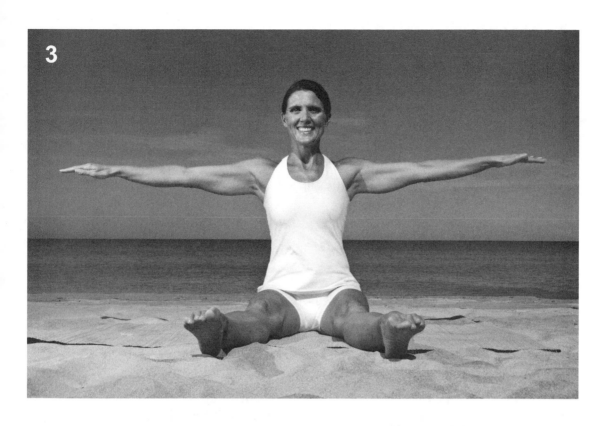

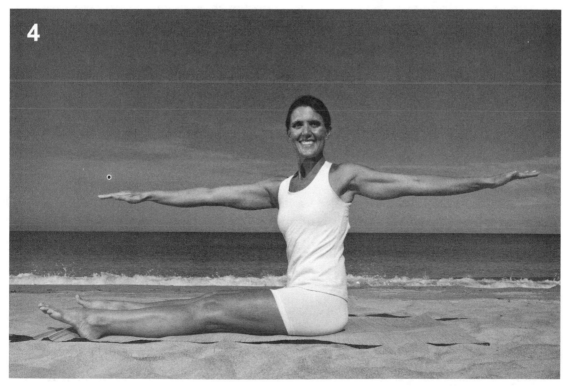

Mermaid

Spinal Movement: Lateral flexion of upper thoracic. Lumbar and pelvic stability.

Step by step:

1. Sitting on your mat, bend the right leg in front of you, left leg reaching behind. You can also sit with both legs crossed in front. The goal is to keep the hips grounded on the mat.
2. Inhale as you extend the arms up to shoulder level, reaching the fingers to opposite ends of the room. Exhale, reach out stretching the spine up and over as you reach your hand down to the floor. Think of the spine long and arched like a rainbow. Keep the hips grounded into the mat feeling the waist lengthen and stretch.
3. Inhale and bring yourself back up to a seated position. Do this by engaging the muscles on the side that is stretching. Use these muscles to lift you back to a seated position.
4. Repeat on the left side.
5. Repeat the movement 4-6 times on each side.
6. Switch the opposite leg in front and repeat.

Pointers for proper execution:

Do move slowly as you focus on lengthening your spine like an arc.
Do breath through every movement, Inhaling and exhaling fully.
Do focus on keeping your abdominals, legs and buttocks active and hips grounded.
Do keep your focus and keep your head aligned with your spine and avoid tilting the head from side to side.

Do not go beyond your range of motion.
Do not let the back arch, shoulders and chin lift.
Do not lift your hips off the mat.

Modifications:

Crisscross the legs in front of you if you cannot reach one leg behind the other. Do not place the hand on the floor if you cannot keep the hips grounded. Always go at your own range of motion and keep the movement small and specific until you gain more flexibility.

How Mermaid helps you during sex:

The unique alternating movement frees up the interaction between the pelvis and the lower spine. Opening the pelvis because of the alternating positions, there is a loosening of the hips while the spine moves gaining better movement for more fluid sexual function.

How Mermaid helps your whole body:

Opening the thoracic spine and rib cage while closing it down on the opposite side is one of the best ways to improve oxygenation and to improve the glide of the nervous system throughout the chest. There is a controlled release and contraction of the pelvic floor, while the deep abdominals control the stability of the pelvis. The piriformes is held in a strong contraction to allow for better independent contraction of the deep transverse abdominus.

Mermaid

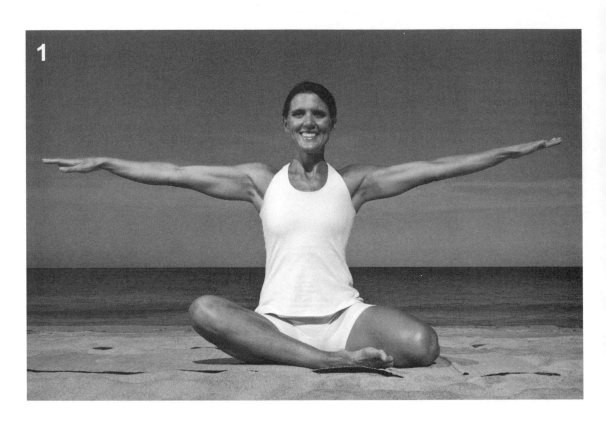

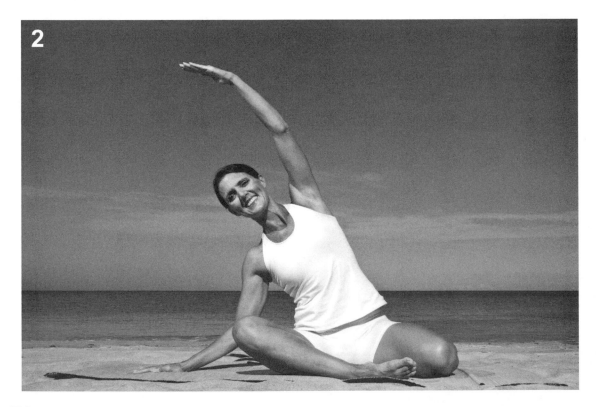

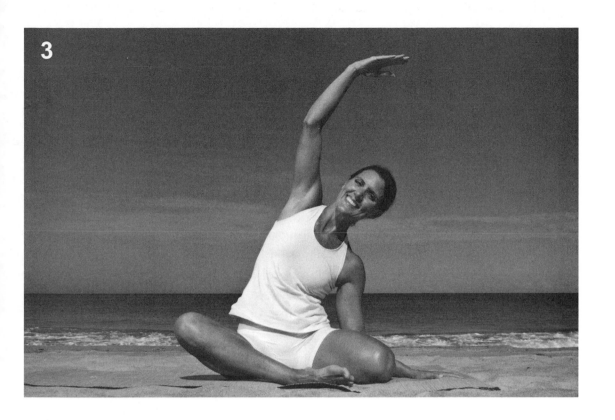

Spinal Wave

Spinal Movement: Full spine articulation, with oscillation of pelvis on the hips.

Step by step:

1. Starting in rest position, knees are hip width apart; arms are shoulder width apart outstretched in front of you on the mat.
2. Exhale, engage the abdominal muscles, lifting them towards your spine.
3. Inhale as you slowly start to move from the tailbone articulating the spine reaching your chest forward. Move fluidly like a wave moving to shore. Come to a tabletop position with the hips over the knees and the shoulders over the wrists. The spine is slightly arched and abdominals active and lifted. Feel the spine long and extended in this position.
4. Exhale as you scoop the pelvis under and round the spine. I like to use the image of an angry cat arching his back. Arms are stretched, tailbone scooped under, head down and abdominals lifted deeper towards the spine as you continue moving back to your rest position.
5. Repeat the whole sequence 5-8 times.

Pointers for proper execution:

Do make sure that your abdominals are active throughout the entire exercise.
Do make sure the hips stay over the knees as you stretch forward.
Do feel as if you are moving through water with very fluid motion.

Do not hyperextend the spine as you come forward.
Do not lift the chin upwards. Keep the head in line with your neck.
Do not hold your breath. If the breath seems too long add extra breaths as you move in order to get full range of motion of the breath and the spine.

Modification:

If you cannot sit all the way back in a rest position stay on all four in a table top position and round the spine and then roll through to a slightly arched back position. Arms stay straight. Hips stay over the knees.
.

How Spinal Wave enhances sex:

Spinal Wave mimics the pelvic motions and control needed for great sex by heavily contracting the hip extensors for good pelvic function. This heavy pelvic contraction aids in full sensual function of the pelvis.

How Spinal Wave helps your entire body:

Spinal Wave loosens the sacroiliac joints rotating them back and forth. There is active lengthening (eccentric) control of the iliopsoas, lengthening where it inserts in the pelvis, grounding it and then lengthening where it attaches in the thigh. The pelvic floor muscles have to work with the surrounding hip muscles and spinal wave trains that action without hundreds of repetitions. Your deepest core muscles begin working while the pelvic floor muscles lengthen. Gliding of the upper lumbar and lower trunk nerve roots both towards and away from the head encourages health for the whole body.

Spinal Wave

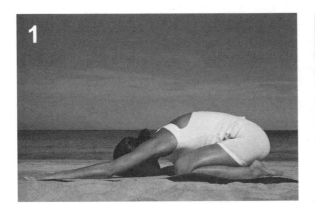

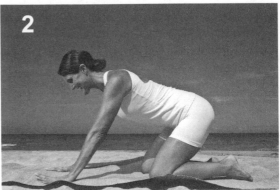

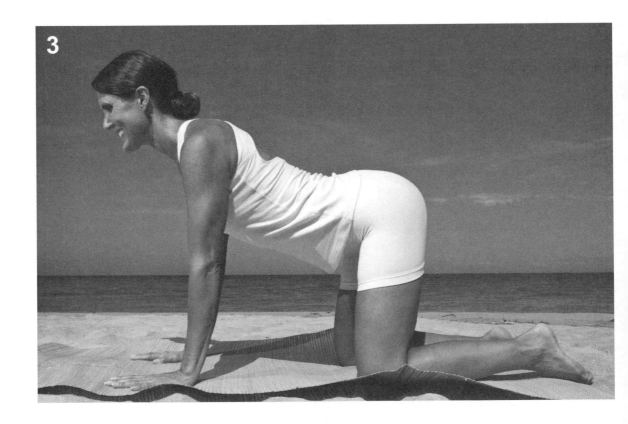

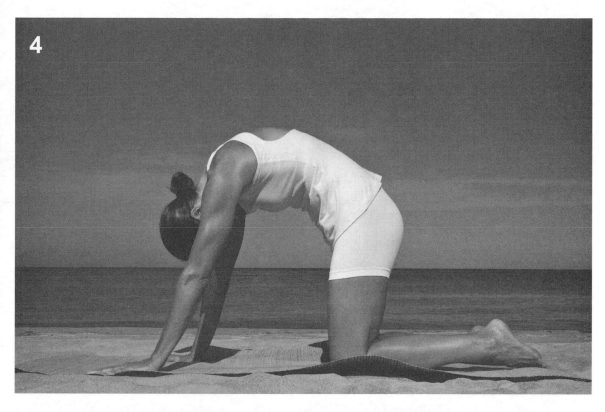

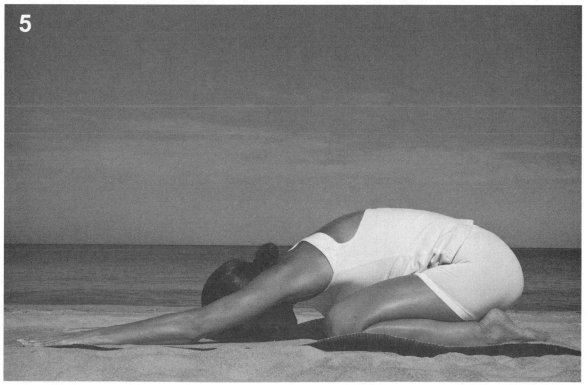

Program #2
(Intermediate)

Program 2 (Intermediate)

By now you and your body should have a better understanding of Pilates and the 8 basic exercises of Program 1. With your daily practice of Program 1, you should have a sense of how the movements feel and relate to your body. You have stayed true and dedicated to your practice and have been on track with Program 1 for 8 weeks. Congratulations! You have probably started to see and feel changes in your body and most importantly your sex life.

The participants of our study noticed an increase in flexibility, strength and over all confidence within the first 8 weeks. They also felt that they had lost some weight and inches and were standing taller and felt leaner overall. In addition, their frequency of sex per week had increased, as did the amount of increased pleasure they found in their sexual experience. Also, for those that were experiencing pain during intercourse before our study noticed a decrease in the amount of pain they felt or the pain completely disappeared. Wonderful results for just 8 weeks of a new Pilates exercise program!

Now that you have mastered Program 1, it is time to begin your new exercises in Program 2. Remember Pilates exercises build on each other and Pilates is a very progressive technique. You will notice with the next series that there are some similarities to Program 1, just a little more challenging. As with any fitness program, if you are not ready to move on, that is fine. Just stay with Program 1 a little longer and progress as you feel ready. Every exercise has a modification so don't be intimidated to try it. Read through the exercises and review the photos to help ease you into the next program. It is not as hard as you think and now that you have a consistent practice with Program 1, you are stronger and more capable than a beginner to move onto Program 2. Always go at your own pace and remember the final goal, a new shapelier, stronger and confident body. In addition, a body and mind that experiences a wonderful and satisfying sexual experience.

The Exercises for Workout 2

Roll-up
Double Leg Stretch
Single Straight Leg Pull
Crisscross
Rolling Like a Ball
Saw
Swan
Side Lying Leg Kick

Roll Up

Spinal Movement: Full spinal flexion, producing neutral and segmental control of each individual vertebra.

Step by step:

1. Lie down on your mat, legs stretched long and hip width apart. Legs are active, feet flexed with toes towards your knees, arms fully extended above your head at shoulder level, fingers reaching to the sky.
2. Inhale as you lower your arms towards your hips slowly peeling the head and shoulders off of the floor.
3. Exhale, engaging the abdominals deeper towards the spine and continue peeling the spine off the mat one vertebra at a time until you reach a hollow C curve position. Reach your hands towards your toes without reaching out of the shoulders. Make sure you reach forward from you abdominals not your arms.
4. Inhale, hold the position. Exhale as you slowly roll back down onto the mat, articulating one vertebra at a time. Reaching the arms above the head at shoulder level to finish, staying active in the body in order to move right into the next roll up.
5. Repeat 5-10 times.

Pointers for proper execution:

Do stay fluid and precise with your movement.
Do keep your head and neck in alignment with the spine.
Do keep your feet grounded so they do not rise off the floor.
Do keep the back muscles active in order to keep the shoulders down and abs engaged.

Do not lean onto one arm to bring yourself up. If you need help hold onto the back of your legs "walking" up your legs to a seated position.
Do not let the shoulders hunch to the ears especially as you roll down.

Modification:

Starting from a seated position, knees slightly bent hold onto the back of the legs and gently guide yourself down, rolling back into a C curve position.   Bend your knees a little more if you need to and do not let the shoulders hunch. You can either roll half way down or all the way down using the hands to guide you, using the abdominal muscles to do most of the work. Roll back up using your abdominals and arms to guide you. Try not to use your hands and arms to bring you up or down and do not lean onto one side. Keep it small and controlled until you gain the strength and proper form in order to move you into full flexion. If this is too hard right now use the Hammock Technique, rolling just the head and shoulders off of the mat.

How Roll Up enhances sex:

Roll Up stabilizes the entire pelvis with a deep co-contraction of the perineum. This is the type of contraction needed for enhanced orgasm. The abdominal muscles contract and lengthen in a rhythmic manner, the use of the inhale, and the exhale improves breathing for sexual intercourse.

How Roll Up helps your entire body:

From a muscle perspective it lengthens structures along the back of the spine, the extensor group, which can tighten through our daily activities like sitting. Roll Up gains wonderful blood flow for the muscles of the hips and the gluteal muscles at the same time the pelvic floor muscles actively lengthen. By grounding the pelvis, the nerve roots from the lumbar spine and the sacrum (tail bone), where they exit the spine, glide against the muscles and bone structures, improving length and function. The repetitive motion of the exercise warms the nervous system in the pelvis and teaches the muscles to release the nerve to improve pelvic function.

Roll Up

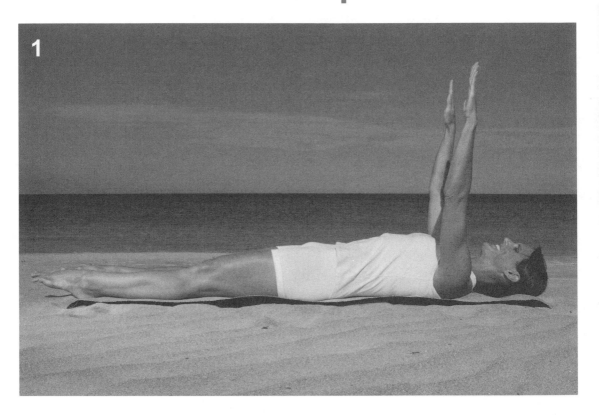

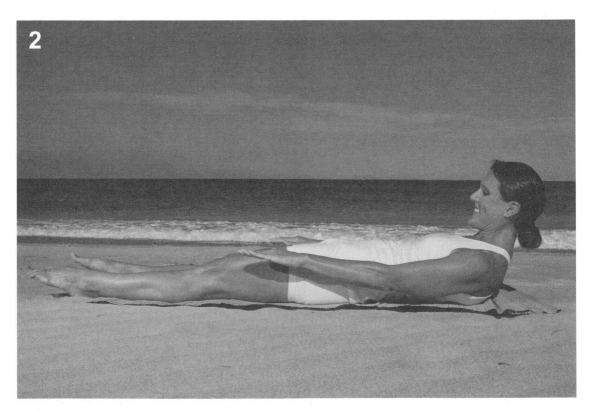

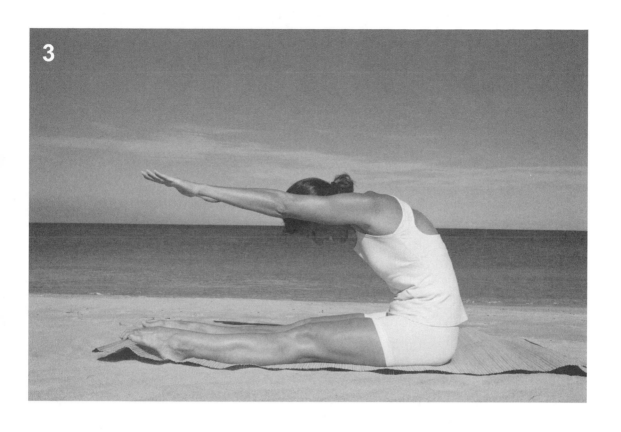

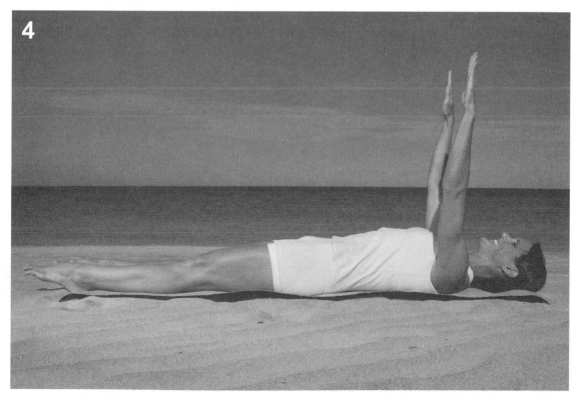

Double Leg Stretch

Spinal Movement: Control and interaction between the pelvic and the sacrum, and stabilization of the lumbar spine.

Step by step:

1. Lie on your back with your knees bent and feet flat on the floor.
2. As you exhale fold your knees into a 90-degree angle. Hold onto the ankles with the hands.
3. Exhale and fold the upper back and head off the mat and into flexion.
4. Inhale, hold the position.
5. Exhale deeply, extending your arms and legs away from your trunk as if someone is pulling you in opposite directions.
6. Inhale come back to your start position, hands on ankles and trunk in flexion.
7. Repeat the arm and leg extension 6-10 times keeping the torso long and neutral without dropping the head or shoulders or arching the back.

Pointers for proper execution:

Do keep your trunk active as you extend the arms and legs.
Do reach the arms and legs actively away from the body.
Do inhale and exhale deeply.
Do keep the back muscles active and strong.

Do not hold your breath.
Do not let your head fall back.
Do not let the back arch.
Do not let the legs drop too low.

Modifications:

If you cannot reach the arms over head without falling back onto the mat keep the hands behind the head and the elbows wide. You can also use the Hammock Technique to help maintain your flexion and just extend the legs. As you get stronger you can lower the legs for an added abdominal challenge.

How Double Leg Stretch enhances sex:

Your quads are a powerful muscle and most noticeably in men there is an imbalance between quads, hamstrings and the hip extensors. This imbalance reduces enjoyment during sex, making it a routine activity and leaving the individual person with low libido. Here you gain a wonderful dynamic balance between these important muscle groups allowing the pelvic floor muscles to function for maximal enjoyment.

How Double Leg Stretch helps your entire body:

Our hip flexors become very tight throughout our day. This exercise actively lengthens them, while the gluteal and pelvic floor muscles contract. The type of contraction gained in the pelvic floor is conducive to greater control of the pelvis during sex, childbirth and other activities involving the pelvis. The nerves in the pelvis glide against the soft tissues of the pelvic floor and against the bone structures while increasing blood flow and range of motion.

Double Leg Stretch

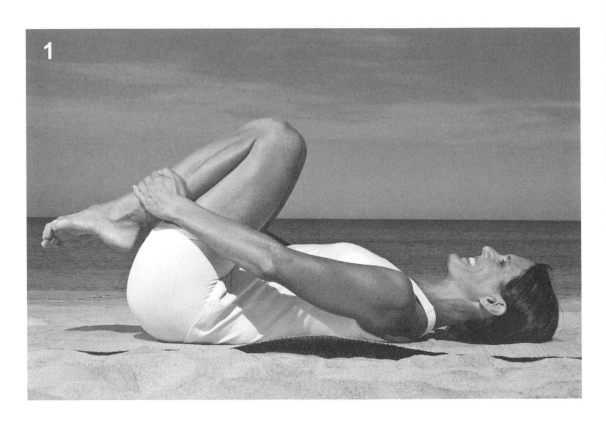

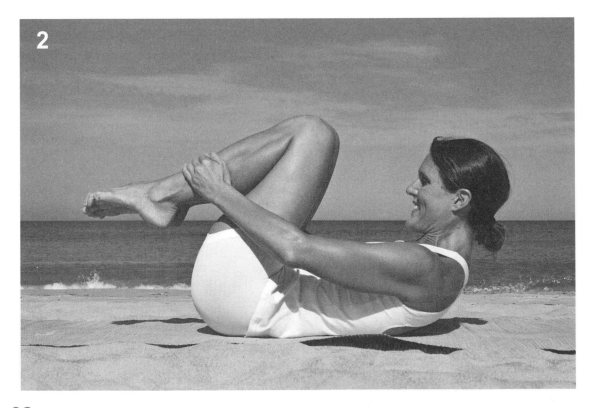

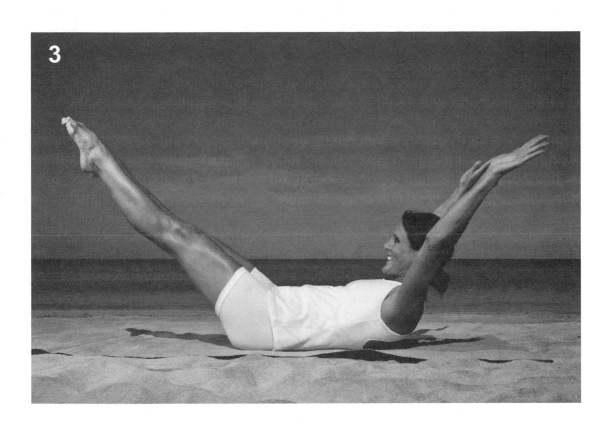

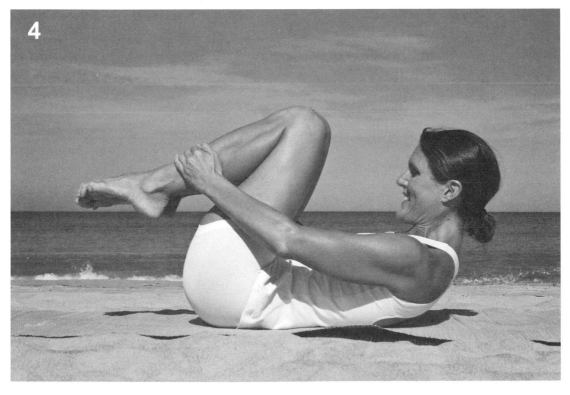

Single Straight Leg Pull

Spinal Movement: Stabilization of the lumbar and sacral region, with dissociation (independent movement) of the hips. Control and stability of each hemisphere of the sacrum while articulating the hips.

Step by step:

1. Lie on your back knees bent and feet flat. Exhale as you fold the knees into a 90-degree angle grabbing onto the ankles.
2. Inhale to prepare.
3. Exhale, fold the trunk into forward flexion.
4. Inhale, straighten both legs into a scissor position, right leg reaching towards the sky and left leg extending from the hip. Depending on your flexibility and range of motion grab a hold of the shin or back of the thigh of the forward leg.
5. Exhale as you draw the right leg towards you with two small pulses feeling a stretch through the leg.
6. Inhale, switch the legs in a scissoring motion reaching through the legs and moving with a stable trunk.
7. Exhale as you draw the left leg towards you with two small pulses, you will feel a stretch through the leg.
8. Inhale, switch legs again and repeat 5-8 times per leg.
9. End by bringing the legs back to your 90-degree angle to finish. Rest.

Pointers for proper execution:

Do use rhythmic breathing and movement.
Do pull the leg towards you in order to stretch the legs.
Do keep your eyes focused on your abdominals.
Do maintain neutral pelvis.
Do keep the abdominals active and hollowing towards the spine.

Do not move too fast and loose the integrity of the movement and position.
Do not let the shoulders hike towards the ears.
Do not pull the leg too much that it pulls your pelvis out of position.

Modifications:

Keep the hands behind the head or use the Hammock Technique. Modify the scissoring motion in order to maintain neutral spine. As you get stronger and more flexible you can make a wider scissor.

How Single Straight Leg Pull enhances sex:

All too often sex becomes boring and routine, and often it is due to lack of ability to perform anything more than the boring positions and repetition that we become used to. This exercise retrains strength in the pelvis while each side functions in opposition to one another. There is extreme stabilization trained in the deep abdominals and the trunk while great eccentric lengthening happens in the perineum creating a wonderful alternating rhythm, preparing you for great sex.

How Single Straight Leg Pull helps your entire body:

Long sliding movements of the legs encourages the sciatic nerve to gain full range of movement while eccentrically (actively) lengthening the hamstrings, gluteals and one side of the pelvic floor muscles and contracting the opposite side. It also encourages rotation of one side of the pelvis while the opposite side is stabilized.

Single Straight Leg Pull

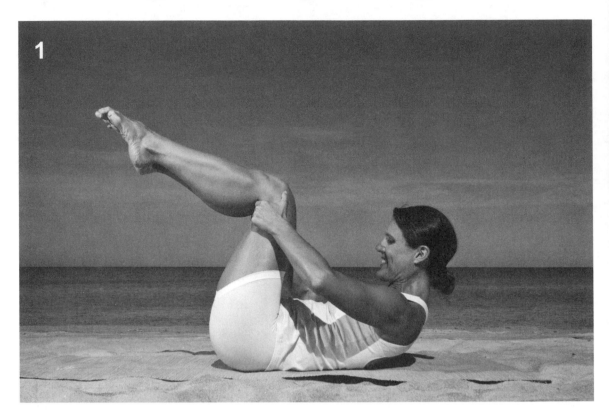

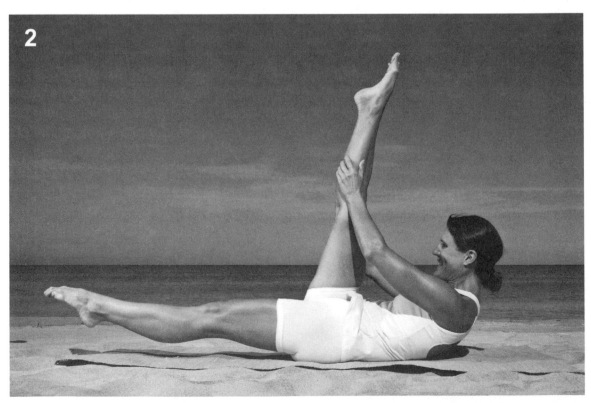

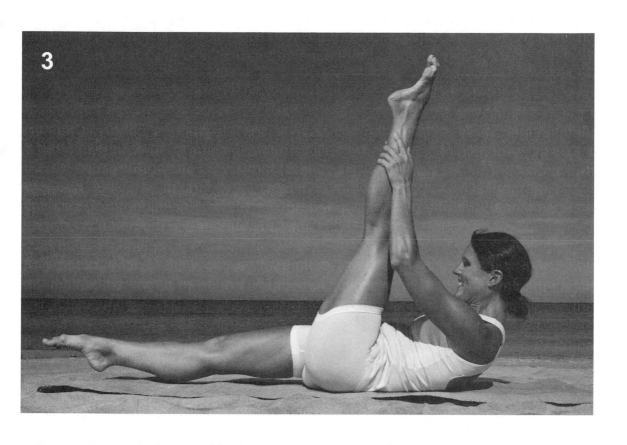

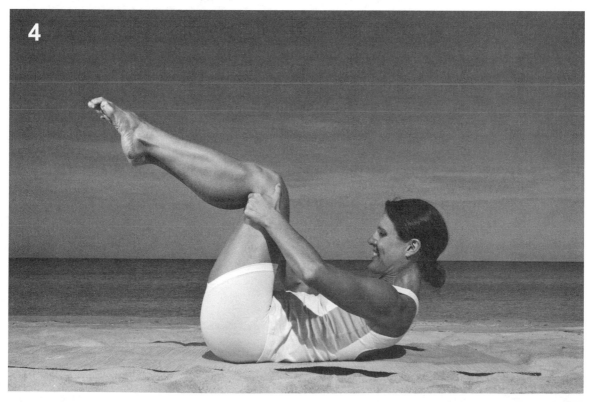

Crisscross (Single Leg Stretch with Rotation)

Spinal Movement: Stabilization of the lumbar column, while rotating the thoracic spine with control.

Step by step:

1.   Lie on your back knees bent and feet flat on the floor. Place your hands behind your head with elbows wide. Exhale and fold the knees into a 90 degree angle.
2.   Inhale and hold the position.
3.   Exhale, fold into flexion maintaining neutral spine.
4.   Inhale and hold the position.
5.   Exhale and extend your right leg out long from the hip and twist towards the left bent knee. Focus on reaching your ribcage to your knee. Your focus is on keeping the elbows wide and looking back towards your elbow to get maximum stretch.
6.   Inhale, return your trunk and legs back to your start position maintaining flexion in the upper trunk. Exhale, extend the left leg as you twist towards the right knee.
7.   Inhale return to center.
8.   Repeat 8-10 times each leg.

Pointers for proper execution:
Do stay in flexion and keep the elbows wide.
Do make sure to look back toward the elbow as you twist to maximize the rotation.
Do keep both hips grounded through the entire exercise.
Do make sure to lead with the ribcage as you rotate.

Do not twist the hips.
Do not bring the elbow to the knee.
Do not let your back arch.
Do not lose the flexion of the trunk when you return to center.

Modifications:

Keep legs higher until you get stronger. If you have trouble staying in flexion keep your head down and don't twist. You can also use the Hammock Technique in order to support the head.

How Crisscross enhances sex:

The obvious answer here would be the oblique muscles, but on closer assessment there is a great complimentary reaction in the small very important pelvic floor muscles. One side gains length with control, while the opposite side shortens in a strong contraction. This is essential for great sex and for those suffering with pain in the pelvic floor, there is great need for this pelvic floor movement to be restored.

How Crisscross helps your entire body:

Here there is wonderful contraction of one side of the pelvis while controlling the opposite oblique and deep core muscles eccentrically (lengthening action). This is so important for normal range of the nerves in the pelvic floor and where they exit from the lower part of the lumbar spine. With Crisscross there is wonderful sliding with improved blood flow to the nerve while the muscles are strengthening for the pelvic floor and the abdominals. Most involved in the hip and back are the hip flexors, which gain great length and the deep core abdominals, which contract and strengthen.

Crisscross (Single Leg Stretch With Rotation)

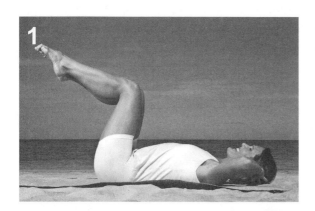

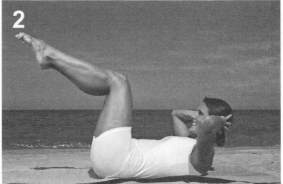

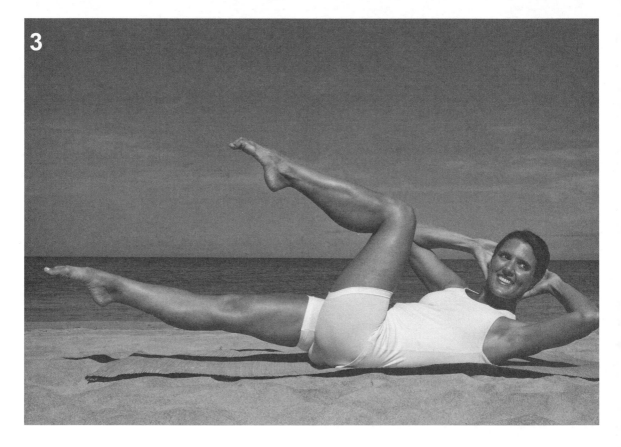

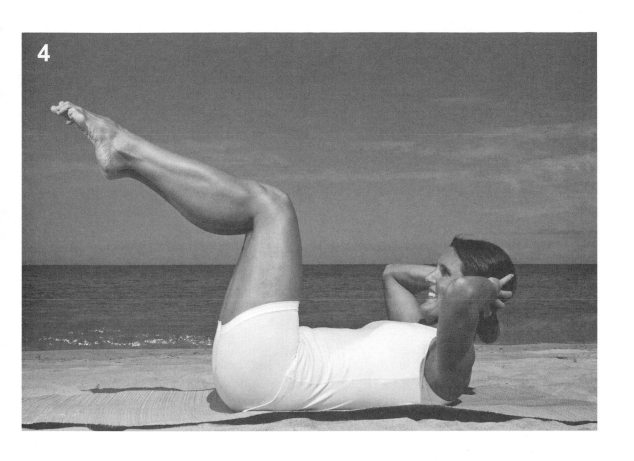

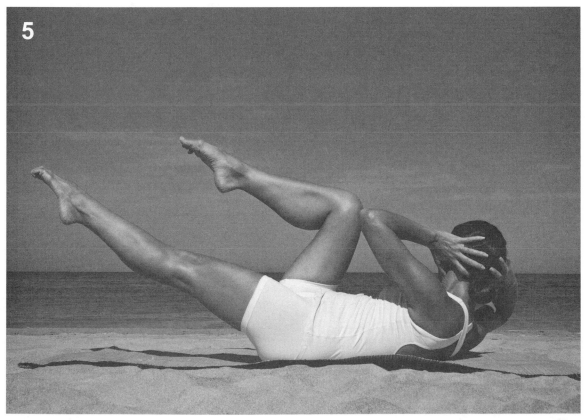

Rolling Like a Ball

Spinal Movement: Full spinal flexion, with massage of the ligamentous structures in the posterior (back) of the spine.

Step by step:

1. Sit towards the front of your mat. Tuck your knees an inch or so from your chest. The knees should be slightly open, feet together.
2. Grab your ankles or just below the knees and round the spine like a ball. Lift your feet off the mat and roll back slightly and balance on your sacrum. The abdominal muscles are active to help you maintain balance and to keep the pelvis tucked.
3. Inhale here to find your balance and prepare for movement.
4. Initiate rolling back by pulling your belly button deep towards your spine as you exhale deeply. You must maintain your round position or you will flatten out like a flat tire.
5. Roll back onto your shoulders, not your neck, with hips high. Exhale deeply as you roll back up to a seated position without touching the mat with your toes. Stop the ball from rolling too far forward by pulling your tummy in deeper. You're ready to roll again!
6. Repeat 8-10 times.

Pointers for proper execution:

Do keep your body round by using your abdominals and back muscles, not your shoulders.
Do keep your shoulders down away from your ears and gaze over your knees.
Do roll to your shoulders keeping your shoulders grounded and away from the ears.
Do stay tight like a ball.

Do not allow your head to fall back, keep your chin tucked.
Do not lead with your head. Lead from your abdominals keeping the spine round.
Do not roll onto your neck.
Do not allow the shoulders to creep up.

Modifications:

Start in the Rolling Like a Ball position lying on your back on the mat this time with your hands behind your knees and elbows wide. Use a little momentum to roll you back and forth till you feel comfortable rolling on your back and up to seated. Now work on rolling without momentum using your abdominal muscles to roll you back and forth and back up to seated. This is a good place to start if you have a fear of rolling back. After a couple of tries you will feel a little more comfortable rolling back onto the mat. If you need to tap your toes for balance when you roll up, do so, but then lift your toes till you are balanced and ready to roll again.

How Rolling Like a Ball enhances sex:

Without the deep abdominals, this exercise is not possible. And there is great rounding of the pelvis, gaining a strong tilt, something absolutely necessary for sex. By tilting the pelvis, sex for both men and women goes from a chore to a pleasure.

How Rolling Like a Ball helps your entire body:

This movement is initiated and sustained by the deep transverse abdominal muscle. While gaining this good contraction – the long hip flexors are elongating to gain full movement. At the same time there is wonderful massage happening to the lower back and pelvis to restore movement where all the nerve roots exit. Those that supply the back and pelvis improve movement and therefore the flow to the pelvic region is improved and so is your sex life!

Rolling Like A Ball

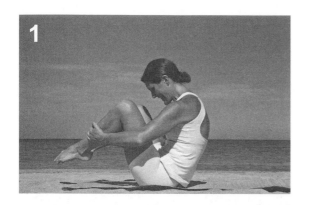

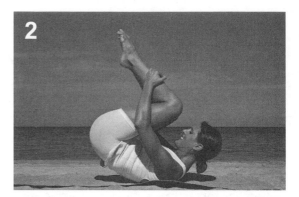

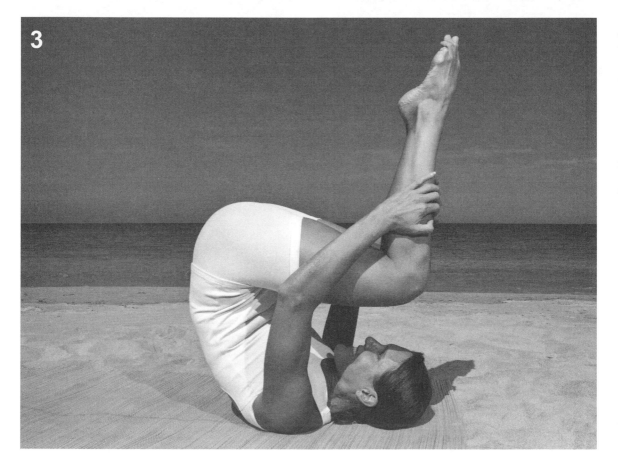

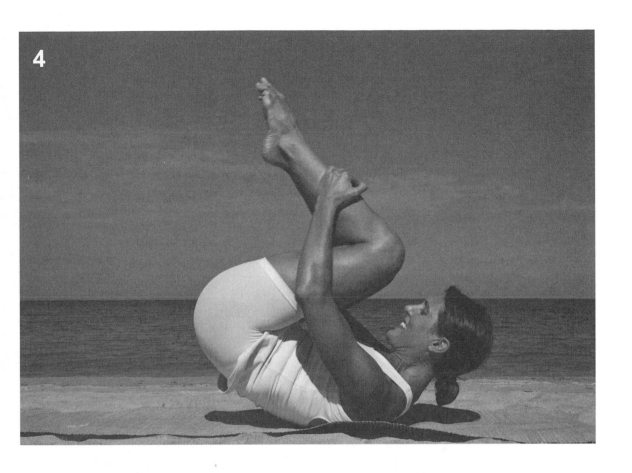

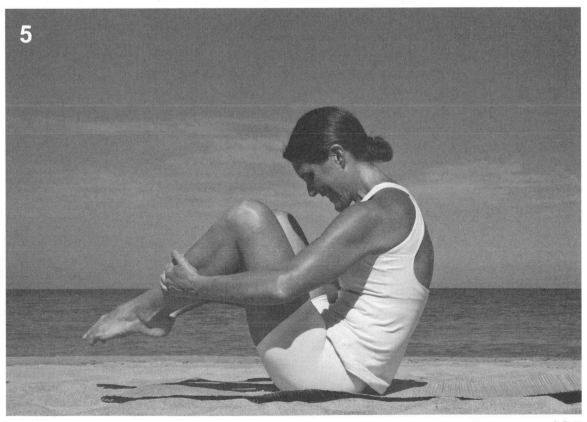

Saw

Spinal Movement: Thoracic rotation and spinal flexion, while stabilizing the pelvis in neutral.

Step by step:

1. Sitting as tall as possible, with the legs wide, about the width of your mat apart, extend the arms reaching to opposite ends of the room. Ground the buttocks into the mat keeping the spine long and straight and feel the ribs float effortlessly above the hips. Imagine a string on the crown of your head being drawn up towards the sky creating length throughout your spine. The abdominal muscles are engaged and active to support the spine.
2. Inhale and twist to the right leg, keeping your hips anchored to the mat. Exhale and round down in a spine stretch position over your right leg. Reach from the abdominals, not from the shoulders. Reach your hand towards your baby toe as if you are sawing off your toe. The opposite arm reaches in the opposite direction.
3. Inhale, roll up to seated still looking towards your foot. Exhale and twist back to your start position making sure your arms are reaching in opposite directions.
4. Repeat on the left side.
5. Inhale, twist left. Exhale, reach long over the leg keeping the opposite hip down, arms are long and extended. Roll back up to a straight seated position looking towards the foot. Exhale and twist back to center.
6. Repeat 5 times on each side.

Pointers for proper execution:

Do keep the hips anchored to the mat as if you are bolted to the earth.
Do keep the shoulders down especially as you stretch towards the leg.
Do initiate movement from your abdominals not from your arms.
Do keep the spine long.
Do imagine your rips floating like a cloud effortlessly off your hips as you sit tall.

Do not let your arms go loose or weak.
Do not allow your shoulders to hunch.
Do not slump in your seated position.

Modifications:

Sit on a pillow, bolster or rolled up mat if you have a hard time sitting tall or if the hamstrings are too tight. The goal is to maintain your position to modify your roll over the leg in order to keep the hips grounded. As you build flexibility you will eventually reach your toes. You can place the hand behind you on the floor to help you maintain position.

How Saw helps your sex life:

The twisting of the pelvis increases the control in the pelvic floor and the lower back, with tensioning of the spine there is increasing control of the small muscles along the spine. The sciatic nerve slides through the hip in a downward direction. This action also increases control in the pelvic floor by alternating active release and contraction. Hamstrings which are so difficult to lengthen, will slowly gain full range, especially since this allows the nerve roots in the pelvis and the lower back to slowly loosen. This gained strength and flexibility will increase your sexual response and allow you to experiment with positions you were may not have tried in the past. OOH la la!!

How Saw helps your entire body:

With grounding of the peripheral nerves, there is wonderful gliding of the nerves through the pelvic structures. The rotation opens the sacroiliac joints with the opposite side compressing for the joint health. And muscles that are really tight in most people, hamstrings and adductors (inner thigh) are wonderfully actively lengthened.

Saw

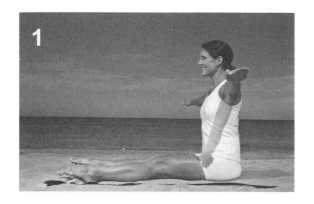

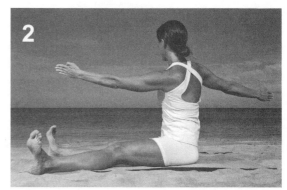

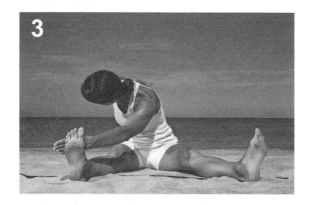

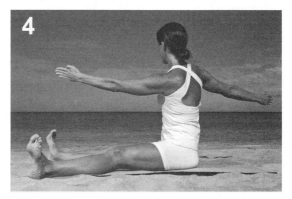

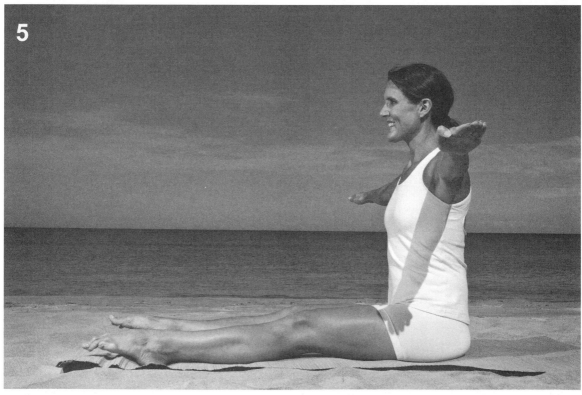

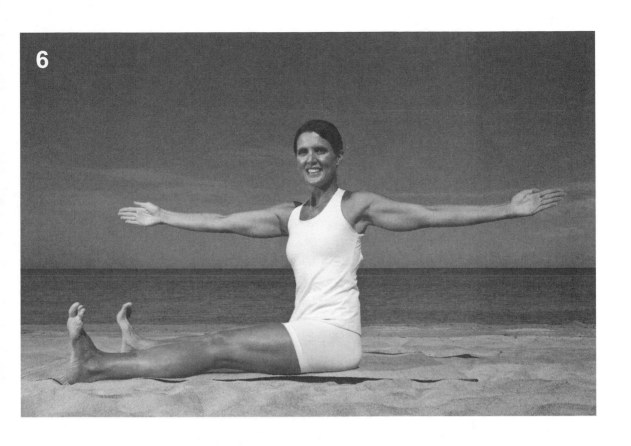

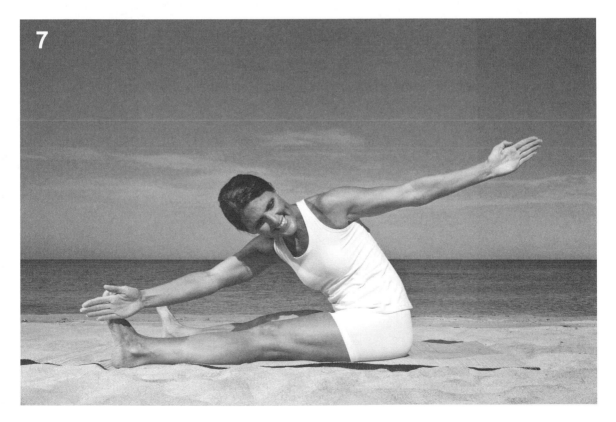

Swan

Spinal Movement: Lumbar, thoracic and cervical extension.

Step by step:

1. Lie on your stomach with the legs reaching back, hip width apart. Arms are bent, hands just below the shoulders.
2. Inhale to prepare.
3. Exhale, pull the abdominals up towards the spine.
4. Inhale again as you slowly rise the chest off of the mat. Make sure to use the extensor muscles of your spine and not your arms to lift you. Your arms will support you but should not do all the work. Keep the hands grounded into the mat. Come up to a comfortable, not forced, back extension.
5. Exhale slowly bring the chest back down to the floor, making sure to stretch the spine as you go forward. Make sure the shoulders never rise towards the ears.
6. Inhale and hold the position.
7. Keeping the upper spine stable and on the mat, exhale and slowly float the legs off of the mat. Keep abdominals active and lifted. Legs are straight. There should be no bend in the knees.
8. Inhale slowly. Lower the legs to the floor.
9. Repeat upper body extension and leg extension 5-8 times, alternating upper body then to lower body.

Pointers for proper execution:

Do press through heels of hands to connect to the sides of the body.
Do pull the abdominals up and in to support the spine.
Do keep your legs straight as if reaching to the back wall.
Do go at your own range of motion.
Do feel the chest lifting as if a harness is pulling you.

Do not force the extension.
Do not sink into the chest and low back.
Do not drop your head back.

Modifications:

Place your hands wider and further away from the body. Float the head and upper back off the mat as if a harness and parachute are pulling you up, but don't come all the way up. Do not lift the legs if it is putting a strain on your back. As you get stronger and more stable you can add the lower body leg lift.

How Swan enhances sex:

The thrill of sex comes with orgasm – and for a strong orgasm the pelvic floor and the adductors of the hips have to be as strong as possible – there is no better way to achieve this than with Swan. While the thighs contract to hold the position there is great release of the abdominals and a co-contraction of the pelvic floor making for stronger control and enjoyment during orgasm.

How Swan helps your entire body:

Swan is great for the discs and all the ligaments anterior (on the front) of the spine. The strength of the back extensors and the length of the big hip flexors have their balance restored. The pelvic floor muscles contract while those same hip flexors give us normal range. Swan improves function in the body and unloads the spinal cord, which is especially good for people that sit a lot.

Swan

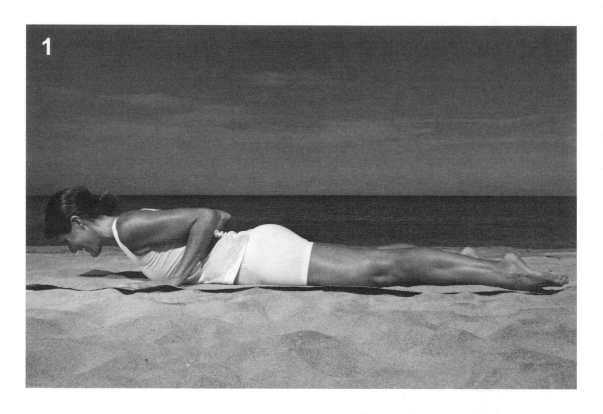

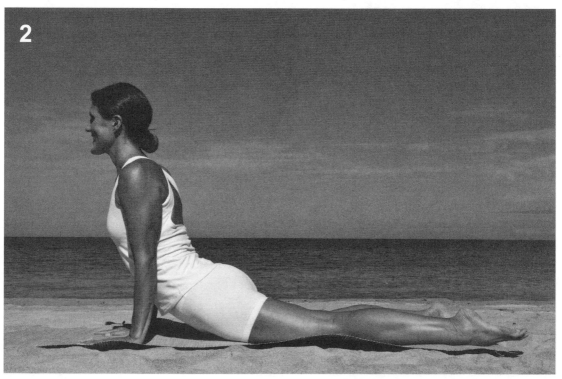

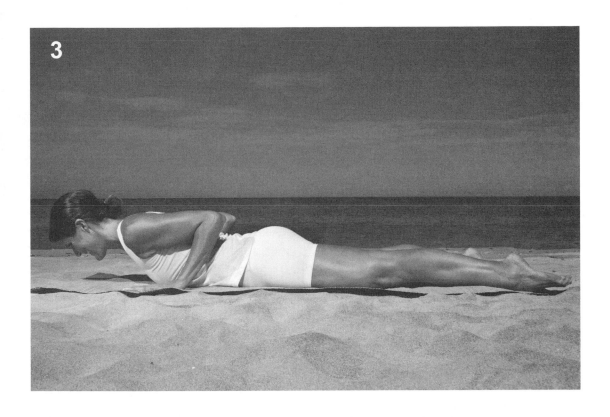

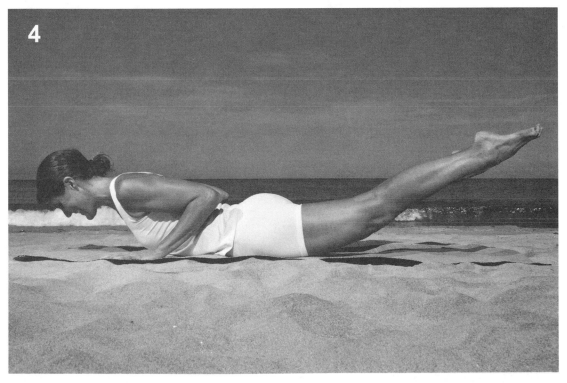

Side Lying Leg Kick

Spinal Movement: Complete spinal stability.

Step by step:

Part 1

1. Lie on your side with your hips stacked and your legs slightly forward in front of you to balance. Rest your head on your outstretched arm. Place the top arm in front of you with the hand on the floor to help you balance and not fall forward. The bottom leg can be bent for more stability or leg long and foot flexed, toes towards the floor.
2. Inhale as you elongate and reach with both legs creating extension through your whole body.
3. Exhale and reach your top leg out in front of you, flexing the foot, toes towards your nose. Keep the spine completely still and long. Feel the back of the leg stretching long out through the heel of the foot.
4. Inhale as you bring the leg back through the center start position.
5. Exhale and reach the leg back away from the body, extending the toes to the wall behind you. The body will want to tip forward here but keep the trunk active to prevent falling forward. The leg should extend behind you at your own range of motion
6. Inhale, bring the leg back to start.
7. Repeat 8-10 times forward and back.

Side Lying Leg Kick - Part 1

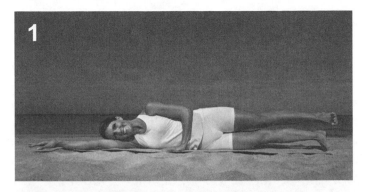

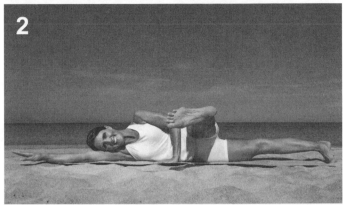

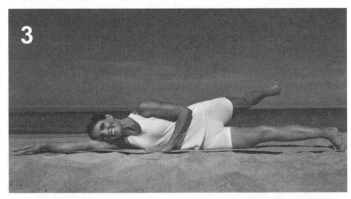

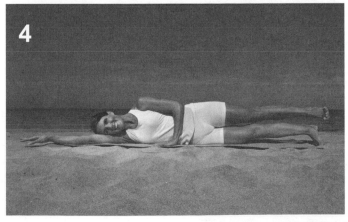

Side Lying Leg Kick

Part 2

Step by step:

1. From the start straight leg position turn the active leg out from the hip so the toes and knee are facing the sky.
2. Kick the leg high reaching the toes towards the sky.
3. Go at your own range of motion keeping the hips bolted together and not swaying side to side. Do not go too high especially if the hips start to fall back or rotate.
4. Flex the foot and squeeze the inner thighs together, reaching the heels towards each other.
5. Repeat 6-8 times.

Turn over and repeat part 1 and 2 on the other side.

Pointers for proper execution:

Do keep your trunk lifted as if you have a harness around your waist lifting you to the sky.
Do keep your abdominals in tight and your ribs knit together.
Do kick only as high as your neutral body will allow.
Do remember the limbs should move freely and independently from the trunk in neutral.
Do breathe!

Do not let your body slouch or fall towards the floor.
Do not kick too far back or forward and compromise the position of the trunk.

Modifications:

Bend the bottom leg for more stability. Bring the legs further out in front of you in a deep "banana" shape. When reaching the leg up in part two, do not go too high and compromise the hip and spine position. Make sure the leg is properly rotated to get maximum range of motion.

How Side Lying Kick enhances sex:

Side Lying Kick exercise is perfect for trunk stabilization while the hips move (hip dissociation). In a side lying position the lateral stabilizers of the spine are recruited and with the rhythmic motion the pelvic floor contracts and relaxes in an orgasmic manner. Perfect balance is required for the abdominals, hips and pelvic floor muscles to work synergistically. As a bonus hamstrings will get longer and leaner for more energetic sex.

How Side Lying Kick helps your entire body:

In the pelvic floor the upper side lengthens actively, while in the lower pelvic hemisphere the pelvic floor muscles contract with the abdominals to stabilize the body. The upper side also allows for active lengthening of tight muscles like the hamstrings and the adductors in the legs, while allowing the sciatic and other important pelvic nerves to glide and lengthen. The foot position encourages all the branches of the nerves, for example the peroneal and tibial nerve in the foot and lower leg to glide as the leg moves.

Side Lying Leg Kick - Part 2

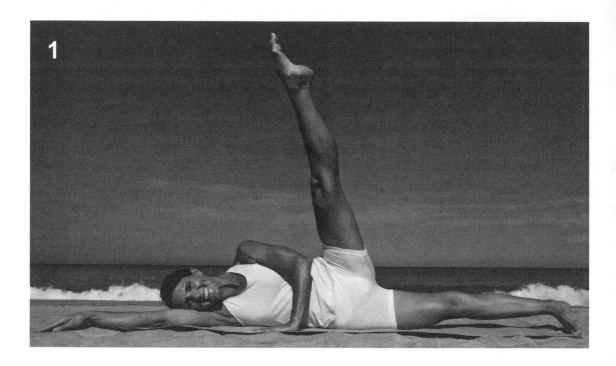

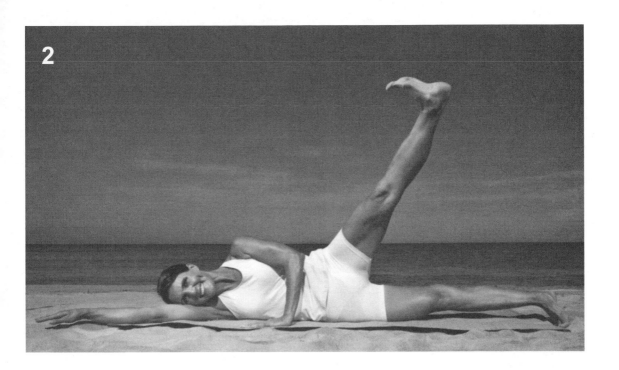

Program #3
(Advanced)

Program 3 (Advanced)

You have made it to Program 3, our most advanced workout. We recommend that you do this program only after you have mastered and executed Program 1 and Program 2 for at least 8 weeks each. If you choose to leap into this program early make sure you use modifications, go at your own pace and listen to your body. This program is intended for advanced practitioners of Pilates.

Program 3 will not only challenge your body but your mind as well. As you have probably noticed in Programs 1 and 2, concentration, coordination and balance of mind body and breath are key to executing a Pilates exercise.

The Exercises for Workout 3

Neck Pull
The Hundred
Pendulum
Roll Over
Open Leg Rocker
Breast Stroke
Double leg kick
Kneeling Side Kick

Neck Pull

Spinal Movement: Full spinal flexion and extension, teaching the spine to remain stable while moving from the pelvis.

Step by step:

1. Lie on your back with your legs straight, hip width apart and feet extended. Place your hands behind your head with elbows wide and slightly lifted off the mat. The muscles of the trunk, abdominals and back should be active and ready to move.
2. Inhale slowly as you roll your chin towards your chest and upper back off the mat. The abdominals draw in deeper towards the spine the elbows are slightly forward and back active.
3. Exhale deeply as you roll the spine off the mat into deep flexion moving one vertebra at a time. Roll the spine into a hollow C curve pressing your legs firmly against the mat.
4. Inhale as you articulate into a straight spine, extending the spine over the legs like a wave rolling and reaching forward. Move fluidly as if moving through water.
5. Lift the lengthened spine to seated, floating the ribs over the hips, with the back long and straight as if sitting against a wall. Do not let the ribs pop out.
6. Exhale deeply as you contract the abdominals and slowly articulate back down onto the mat, one vertebra at a time, keeping the abdominals active and shoulders down away from the ears.
7. Repeat 6-8 times.

Pointers for proper execution:

Do keep the shoulders down away from your ears to keep the back muscles active.
Do keep the legs active and pressing into the mat.
Do stay focused on rolling up through the center. Stay balanced using the back and the abdominals to do so.

Do not pull the neck too hard and drop the chin to the chest.
Do not lean on one arm or the other to get up. Modify till you get stronger.
Do not let the legs come off the floor.

Modification:

If you cannot roll up with the hands behind the head, roll up as if you are doing the Roll Up exercise with hands reaching out in front of you. You can also walk the hands up the legs to get you to a seated position. When you come to a seated position place the hands behind the head. Continue rolling into a seated C curve position. Continue extending the spine to a tall seated position before you start to roll back down. Release the hands again in order to help you roll back down to your start position on the mat.

How Neck Pull enhances sex:

With the legs well grounded, hamstrings have to use their full length and the spine has to round with fluidity – this lithe action is the perfect way to create sensual sexual movement. The abdominal muscles contract strongly to move the entire torso. Their interaction with the hip extensors and those big gluteals allow for more flexibility and strength at the end of that enhanced range – taking sex to the next sensual level.

How Neck Pull helps your entire body:

The rolling motion loosens the sacroiliac and lumbar joints, with a massaging action to the long ligaments and muscles in the back. With the segmental movement of each vertebra it improves the slide of all the nerve roots as they exit the spine and the sacrum. The nerves get oscillating change in blood flow and range, which improves their function. During the rolling up there is deep contraction of transverse abdominus – producing stability for the back and good antagonistic support for the pelvic floor muscles

Neck Pull

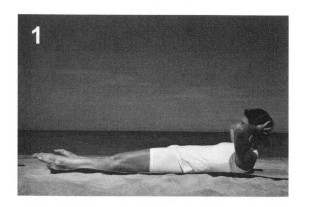

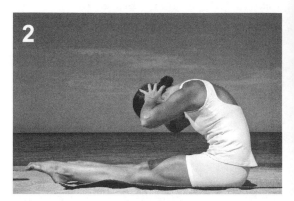

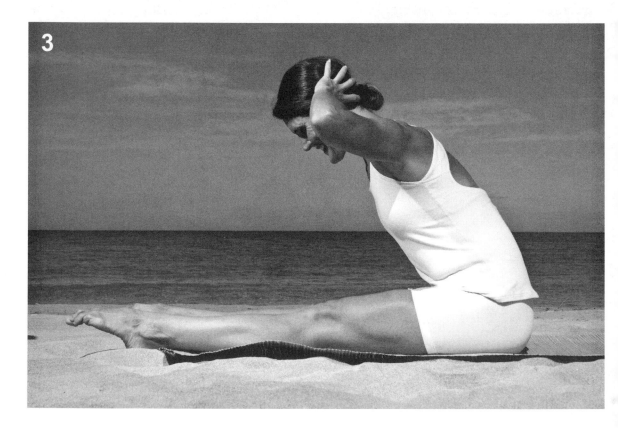

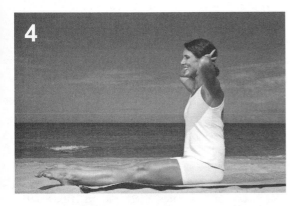

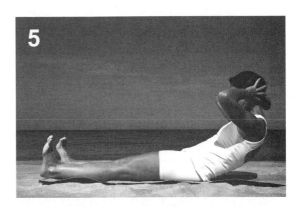

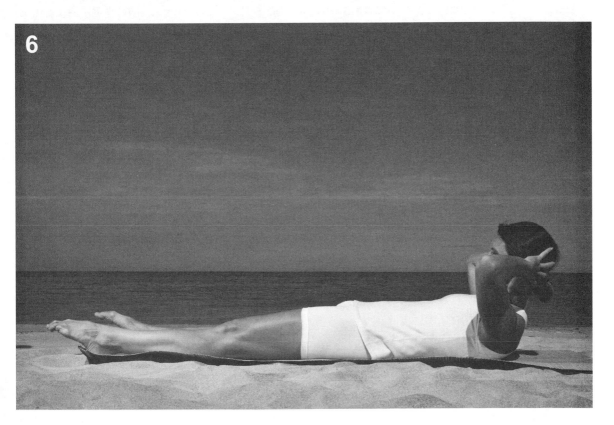

The Hundred

Spinal Movement: Flexion of the thoracic and cervical spine, controlling the pelvic position to gain optimal function in the deep abdominals.

Step by step:

1. Lie on your back with knees bent, feet flat on the mat.
2. Exhale and fold the knees into a 90-degree angle, placing the hands on the ankles.
3. Inhale and hold the position.
4. Exhale as you bring the upper trunk into flexion. Release the arms and reach them long with fingers towards the end of the mat. The sternum is relaxed and shoulders down away from the ears. Legs reach at a diagonal away from the center of the body, maintaining the integrity of the back and abdominals
5. Pump the arms up and down vigorously. Only move the arms and keep the shoulders stable. The goal is to develop a pumping type breath (diaphragmatic breathing) of 5 quick inhales and 5 quick exhales for a total of ten breaths. Ten breaths equal one set. Repeat 10 times for a total of 100.
6. After set 10 inhale stop the arms and hold the position. Exhale and fold the knees to the chest lower the head and shoulders and rest.

Pointers for proper execution:

Do go slowly at first gradually building strength and stamina.
Do count your breaths.
Do keep your focus on your abdominals.
Do be patient and work up to 100 breaths gradually. You did the Hundred Modified the first 8 weeks so it should feel familiar and easier, but still go at your own pace.

Do not let your shoulders hike to your ears.
Do not compromise on form or breath to get to 100.
Do not hold your breath!

Modifications:

Keep knees bent and feet on the floor. Keep head down or use the Hammock Technique to help yourself up. Modify the breathing by taking long breaths in and out. Work up to 5 by starting at 2 or 3 pulses and so on.

How The Hundred enhances sex:

Moving to the next level, when you have been doing the exercises for 16 weeks or more this will warm the deepest layer of the abdominals with a strong contraction of the pelvis. The intense warming is what we need for pleasurable sex, in addition to strengthening the hip rotator and extensors – which lead to a more powerful sexual experience.

How The Hundred helps your entire body:

The Hundred creates deep abdominal and core strengthening, and increases the stabilization function in the pelvic floor. The small oscillations warm the entire nervous system, improving blood flow and allowing for great gliding of the nerves against the muscles and joints. The breathing is important – muscles and nerves will not remember movements as easily as they do when they are starved for oxygen and here we immediately create great blood flow and oxygen for the entire body.

Hundred

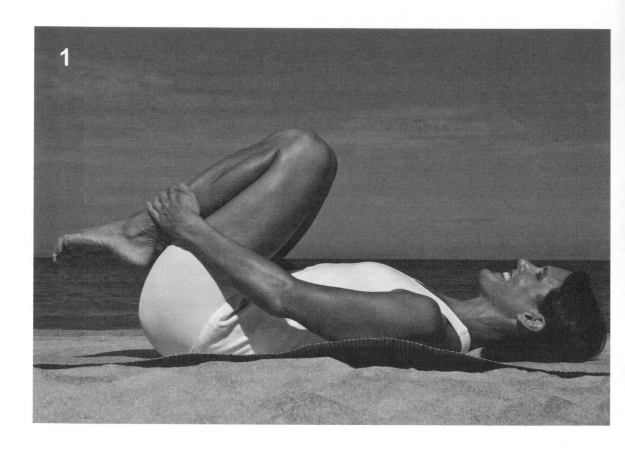

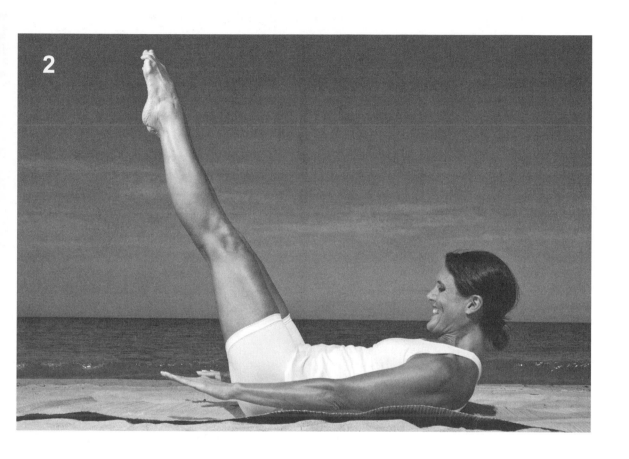

Pendulum

Spinal Movement: Lumbar rotation and controlled thoracic dynamic stability.

Step by step:

1. Lye on your back knees bent and feet flat. Arms are stretched out in a T position from the shoulders for upper trunk stability.
2. Exhale and fold the knees into a 90 degree angle and extend at the knees to a straight leg position reaching from the hips to the sky. Spine is neutral and pelvis is neutral.
3. Imagine a marble in the belly button. As you inhale slowly roll the marble to the left hip (or 3 o'clock position) twisting from the waist lifting the right hip off the mat, reaching the legs long
4. Exhale deeply and slowly, rolling the hips and legs back to the start position. Initiate the movement from your abdominals and not your back. Imagine the marble rolling back to the belly button, finding neutral again.
5. Repeat on the right side rolling the marble to the 9 o'clock position.
6. Inhale, return to center.
7. Repeat 6-8 times on each side.

Pointers for proper execution:

Do keep your head in line with your spine at all times.
Do keep the shoulders grounded and away from the ears.
Do keep your gaze up and the head still.
Do maintain length through the spine at all times.

Do not let the shoulders come off of the floor.
Do not let the tailbone roll off the mat when you are centered and neutral.
Do not lift the hip towards the armpit.

Modification:

Bend the knees into a 90 degree angle keeping the feet in line with the knees.

How Pendulum enhances sex:

In Pendulum the perineum and hip muscles are guided and strengthened for contraction during orgasm. The abdominals contract and eccentrically release for greater pelvic control during sex.

How Pendulum helps your entire body:

The side-to-side motion loosens the sacroiliac joint and the lumbosacral joints.

There are synergistic actions between the abdominals and the pelvic floor, which is what we need for daily function, and at the same time there is deep core stabilization occurring. The "wringing out" that occurs in the abdominals is important as it encourages pelvic floor control as the pelvis rocks. The large sciatic nerve glides across the hips while the branches that terminate in the foot are anchored, encouraging maximal glide through the hip and the pelvis.

Pendulum

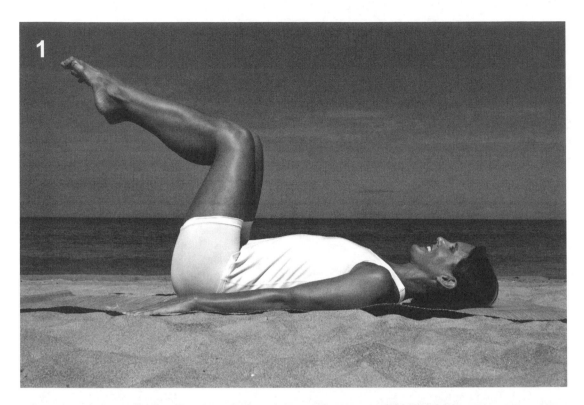

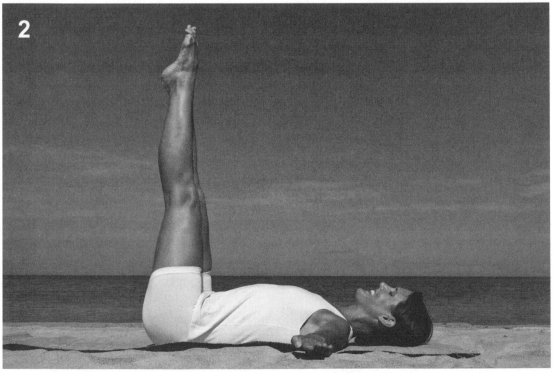

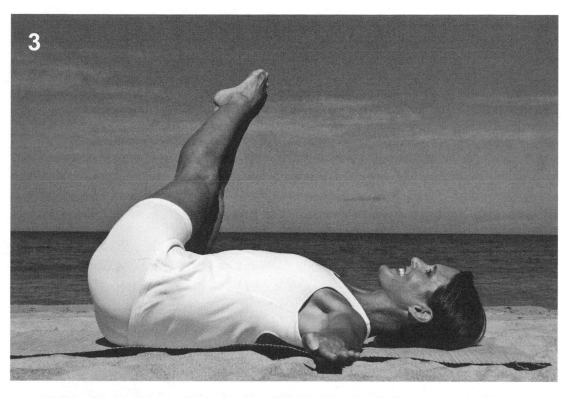

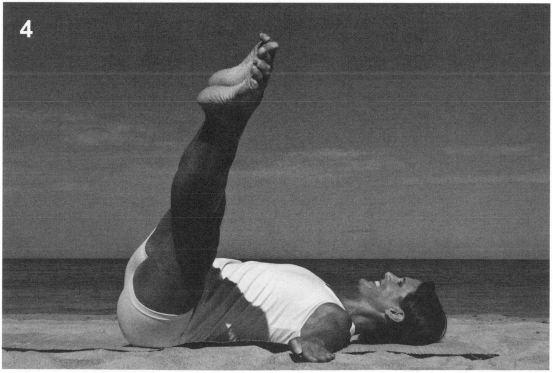

Roll Over

Spinal Movement: Full spinal articulation with an extraordinary amount of range from the sacroiliac joints.

Step by step:

1. Lie on your back knees bent, arms reaching long along the body.
2. Exhale as you fold your knees into a 90-degree angle and extend your legs out to a diagonal grounding your hips and keeping the arms active and long.
3. Inhale and bring the legs straight up in line with the hips.
4. Exhale deeply, using the abdominals, peel the spine off the mat one vertebra at a time bringing the hips above the shoulders and feet towards the floor behind you.
5. Stretch the legs over the head keeping the legs long and active. Balance on your shoulders (not your neck).
6. Flex the feet and separate the legs, hip width apart, for the roll down.
7. Inhale as you slowly begin your roll down off of the shoulders. Then exhale fully as you continue the roll down, one vertebra at a time, through the mid back, lower back and hips, continuing to your start position. The abdominals and back muscles are actively guiding you down with control and precision. Allow your arms to reach with you as you stretch the spine back down onto the mat, keeping the shoulders and mid back from hunching.
8. Repeat 6-8 times.

Pointers for proper execution:

Do keep your head and shoulders down during the whole exercise.
Do keep the legs straight.
Do allow the spine to move fluidly executing the movement from your abdominals and back muscles.
Do use your arms to help ground your upper trunk but do not use the arms to push you over.

Do not let your shoulders hike towards your ears.
Do not let your head lift.
Do not use momentum to roll over.
Do not roll onto your neck.

Modification:

If you do not want to attempt Roll Over or have back or neck issues you can do Bridging (from Workout 1). If you do not have the strength to get yourself over, use a bolster, rolled up mat or towel to prop up your hips. This will give your hips a little lift to get started. Using your breath and your lower abdominals slowly roll and lift your hips off of your support reaching your feet towards the floor behind your head.

How Roll Over enhances sex:

This is so much more than an abdominal exercise. Roll over creates an incredibly deep abdominal contraction and lengthening of the big gluteals (butt muscles). This helps reduce fat content, lengthening and leading to a sexier leaner muscle. There is also a strong eccentric contraction of the pelvic floor for both men and women – improving the pleasure of the sexual experience, most noticeable in those people who suffer with pain during sex.

How Roll Over helps your entire body:

This is how you can tension and glide the entire nervous system, encouraging glide of the nerves through the sacrum as you roll down onto it, opening both sacral joints. There is also eccentric control gained from the pelvic floor in balance with the need for good deep core control. The rolling produces great massaging action of the entire posterior spine.

Roll Over

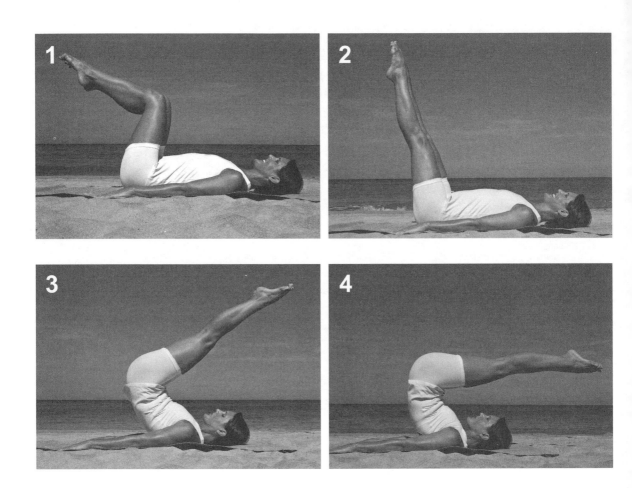

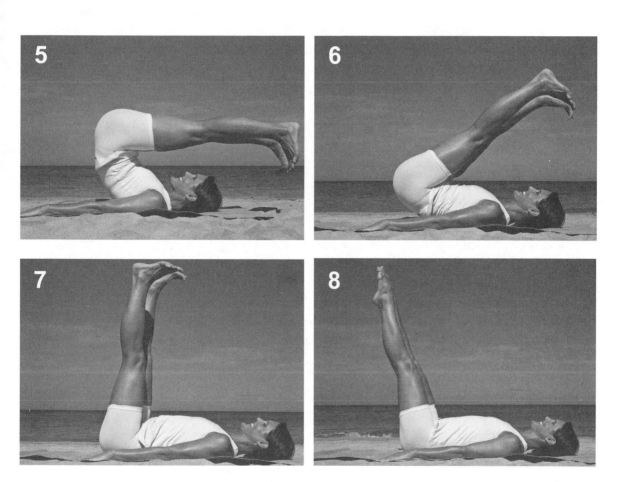

Open Leg Rocker

Spinal Movement: Sacroiliac control and gapping, (opening and closing of the sacroiliac joints), while gaining spinal flexion and extension in measured amounts.

Step by step:

Part 1

1. Balancing on your buttocks, bend your knees towards you and hold onto the back of the knees. Knees and feet are hip width apart and are parallel with the hips. The spine is long and straight.
2. Exhale and straighten both legs upward and then outward to a V position, shoulder width apart.
3. Inhale bend back to the bent knee position.
4. Repeat this 5 times for breath and balance.

Part 2

As you master the balance, add a roll back and back up.
1. With legs fully extended exhale deeply to initiate you're rolling by pulling the abdominals deeper towards the spine and scooping the pelvis. This in turn pulls you off balance.
2. Roll back with control balancing on your shoulders without dropping the feet to the floor behind you. Keep the spine long and hips lifting as you roll back, balancing onto your shoulders.
3. Exhale as you pull the abdominal muscles in deeper keeping the spine round. With control, roll back up to your seated balance.
4. Repeat 5-8 times.

Pointers for proper execution:

Do keep your trunk tall and do not hunch in the shoulders.
Do roll with control, like your moving through water.
Do balance on your shoulders and keep your hips high when you are in your roll back position.
Do bring the hands lower down the legs if you cannot balance or you find that your shoulders hunch.
Do soften the knees if your legs are tight and if you cannot maintain a long spine.

Do not roll down further than you can roll up.
Do not lead with your head. If you throw your head back you will "flatten" like a flat tire. Maintain your round back position in order to roll up to your balance.
Do not hunch the shoulders or round the upper back.
Modifications:

Keep your knees bent and in line with your feet as you roll. As you get stronger, gain more balance, flexibility and control, you can lengthen the legs long. If you are not ready to roll back practice the balance and breathing for a few days until you feel more comfortable and confident.

How Open Leg Rocker enhances sex:

The iliopsoas is one of the most important hip flexors muscles since it bridges abdominal and hip function. The ilipsoas needs to be strong, supple and powerful for an enhanced sexual experience. Open Leg Rocker builds that strength and suppleness in the iliopsoas for enhanced sexual pleasure and a less painful sexual experience.

How Open Leg Rocker helps the entire body:

There is eccentric control of the pelvic floor muscles while the core structures are initiating movement. This is what allows our pelvis to return to normal function and it allows activities like sex to be pain free. The wide leg position of the hips, tensions up additional branches of sciatic and obturator nerves. The nerves are massaged with the rolling action and gliding across the hips, while their roots in the spine are loosened up significantly.

Open Leg Rocker

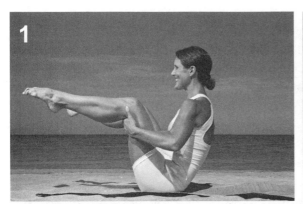

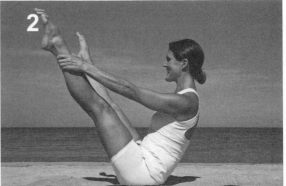

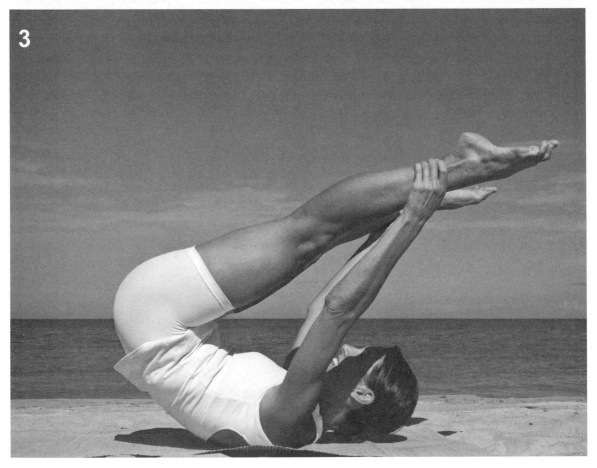

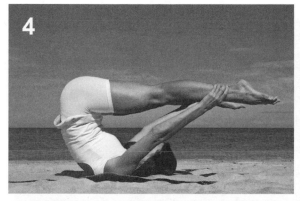

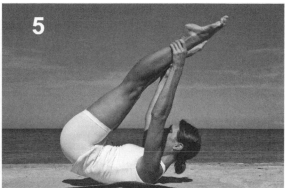

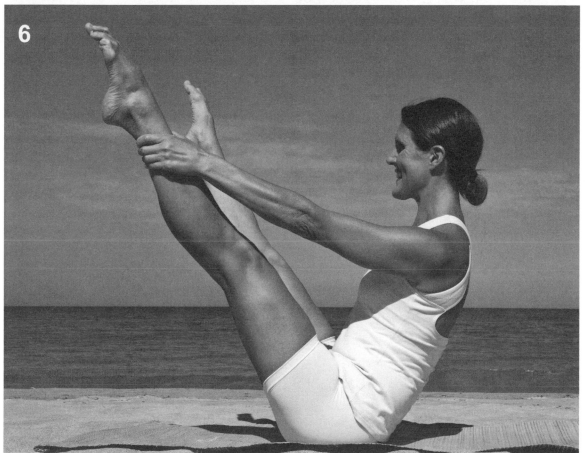

Breast Stroke

Spinal Movement: Initial lumbar extension, with thoracic and cervical extension being added

Step by step:

1. Lie on your stomach, completely outstretched on the mat. Bend your arms by your side, hands by your armpits.
2. Exhale as you extend through your legs and back. Activate and lift the abdominal muscles towards the spine.
3. Inhale as you reach your arms straight out in front of you, beyond the mat. Feel the arms extend from your back keeping the shoulders down away from the ears.
4. Exhale as you sweep your straight arms away from each other, extending the upper trunk and legs off the floor. Sweep your arms all the way around reaching your fingers to your feet.
5. Inhale as you bend the elbows bringing the hands back to your shoulders and through the start position. Continue breathing as you move right into the next repetition.
6. Repeat 5-8 times.

Pointers for proper execution:

Do stay long and extended with your arms and legs.
Do keep your abdominals lifted and active throughout the exercise.
Do feel as if you are moving through water.
Do keep the arms active and extending from the back.

Do not hunch the shoulders towards the ears.
Do not let the abdominals go weak.
Do not rest in between repetitions.
Do not hold your breath!

Modifications:

Keep the legs on the floor throughout the movement but keep them active and grounded into your mat. If you need to rest in between each repetition please do so, then continue onto the next movement after your short rest.

How Breast Stroke enhances sex:

Creating a long lean lower back and butt can only improve your sex life. Also, creating length out of the tight hip flexors can help reduce pain. Hamstrings hold tight to stabilize the hips, while the lower abdominals contract for strength and stability.

How Breast Stroke helps your entire body:

The extended position unloads the spine, improves the nutrition to the discs between each vertebra and places the nerve roots in a low load position. Through the exercise there is gliding of the femoral nerve across the front of the hip. The iliopsoas muscle and the anterior abdominal muscles have to work eccentrically, while the pelvic floor contracts with the transverse abdominus – this dynamic action is how we can optimize pelvic function.

Breast Stroke

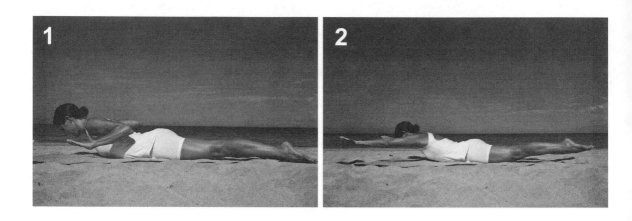

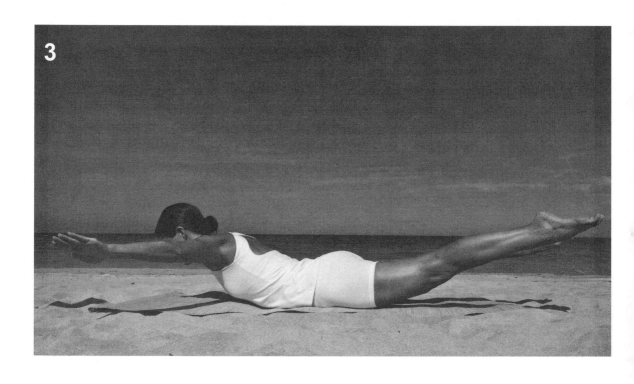

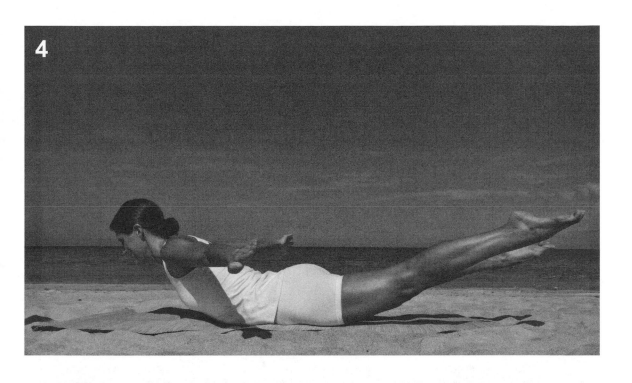

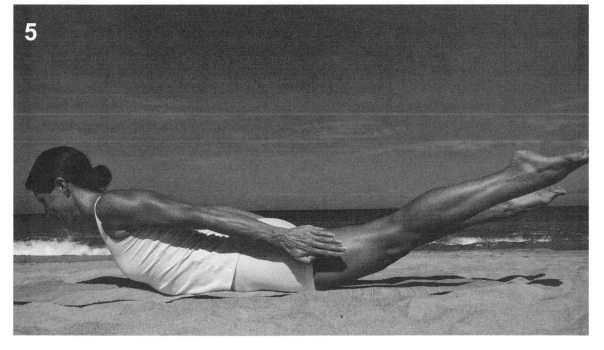

Double Leg Kick

Spinal Movement: Lumbar extension, with added thoracic and cervical extension, while stabilizing pelvic position

Step by step:

1. Lie on your stomach with your head facing one side. Clasp your hands behind your back and place them as high up your back as is comfortable. Make sure the front of your elbows and shoulders are relaxed on the mat.
2. Squeeze your buttocks and inner thighs together. With 3 quick exhales kick both heels to your buttocks, three times. Feet are flexed and the emphasis is on the heels to the buttocks.
3. Inhale, rotate the head to neutral, extend the legs and bring the upper trunk into extension as the arms extend behind you reaching towards the legs. The back muscles are active and strong. Feel as if you are floating off the mat, crown of the head and legs extending in opposite directions. The whole body is active and energized.
4. Exhale, return to the original kicking position, body lying on the mat, head facing opposite direction and hands clasped as high up the back as possible. Let the head, shoulders and elbows relax as you kick the heels to the butt three times with three quick exhales.
5. Inhale and extend the body long and lean again, feeling as if you are floating off the mat arms and legs extending, the crown of the head reaching in the opposite direction.
6. Exhale and come back to your start position
7. Repeat 6-8 times.

Pointers for proper execution:

Do make sure the arms are reaching long behind you.
Do try to reach them past your buttocks.
Do keep the abdominals pulling up to the spine throughout the exercise to support your lower back.
Do make sure to rotate the head side to side with each interval.

Do not allow your buttocks to lift as you kick your heels to the buttocks.
Do not hunch the shoulders towards the ears.
Do not lift the chin while you extend the spine. Head stays long and neutral.

Modifications:

If you have tight shoulders and cannot reach your hands together keep the arms extended by your side. If you do not want to lift the legs keep them stretched on the floor after you kick and come into your spine extension.

How Double Leg Kick enhances sex:

To improve on the strength you have created over the past few weeks, this takes you to the next level of improved hip strength and deep abdominal control. Heightening the experience of sex taking it to the next level of pleasure, by boosting your strength and control in the pelvis and the perineum.

How Double Leg Kick helps your entire body:

There is great extension of the lumbar spine, anterior rotation of the sacrum, with a good co-contraction of the hips, pelvic floor and the core structures; you gain eccentric length in the hamstrings and the rectus abdominals (getting us a better looking six pack!). The femoral nerve which runs along the front of the thigh, slides against the quads gaining range and a long lean, sexy muscle!

Double Leg Kick

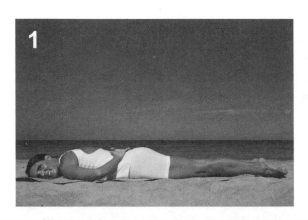

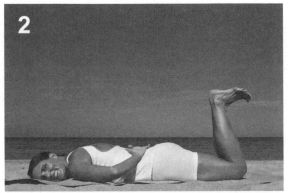

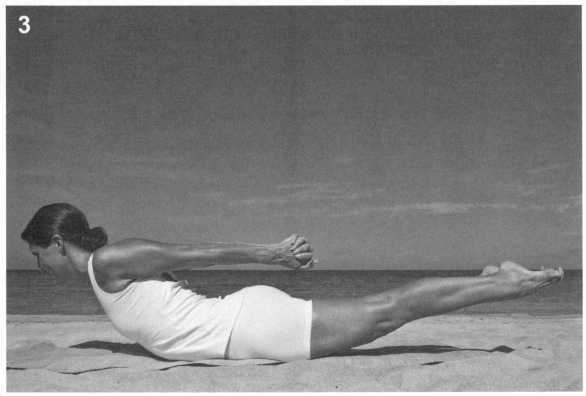

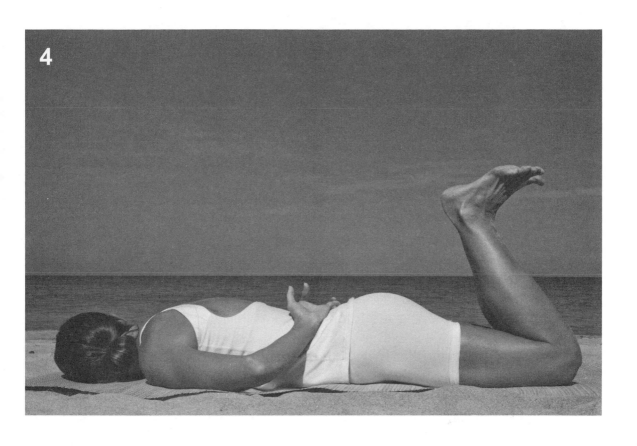

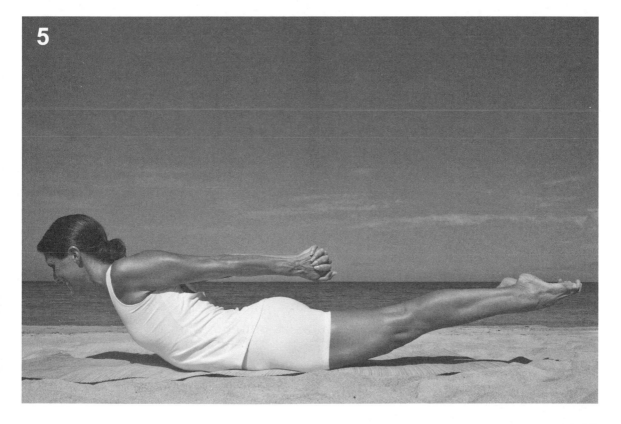

Kneeling Side Kick

Spinal Movement: Control and stability of the pelvis and entire spine, with the unique position of the pelvis this enhances the stability and function of the sacrum with hips spread during movement.

Step by step:

1. Kneel on your mat and prop yourself up on one hand. Make sure the arm is aligned directly beneath your shoulder. Place your opposite hand on your hip or behind your head. Do not let the shoulder roll forward.
2. Inhale as you lift your top leg into the air to hip height. Turn the leg out slightly to engage the buttocks. Stabilize your shoulders, hips and trunk. Do not allow any movement except from the extended leg.
3. Exhale, reach the leg out in front of you extending from the back of the leg reaching long through the heel. Go at your own range of motion and do not compensate by letting the trunk lose its stability or neutral position. Keep the trunk active.
4. Inhale as you bring the leg back through the center beginning point. Continue extending the leg back behind you, maintaining integrity of the neutral spine.
5. Continue the motion forward and back, repeating 5-8 times on each leg.

Pointers for proper execution:

Do keep active in your waistline to help take pressure off the supporting wrist.
Do keep a slight turnout in your leg to work your buttocks and the back of the thigh.
Do stay square in your body making sure to keep your hip directly over the bent knee.
Do continually deepen the scoop in your trunk while pushing the pubic bone forward.
Do keep the crown of your head reaching in the opposite direction of your extend leg.

Do not fall into the supporting arm.
Do not shorten the spine by hunching or slouching in the trunk.
Do not lose the integrity of the abdominals.

Modifications:

If you are not ready for Kneeling Side Kick, have wrist issues or just don't feel strong enough yet then do side Lying Leg Kick from Program 2.

How Kneeling Side Kick enhances sex:

This exercise is perfect for trunk stabilization while the hips move (hip dissociation). And because you are balancing on one hand and knee, the lateral stabilizers of the spine are recruited. With the rhythmic motion the pelvic floor contracts and relaxes in an orgasmic manner. The advanced positioning improves the deep pelvic stability and pelvic floor control. As a bonus, the hamstrings will just get longer and leaner for more energetic sex.

How Kneeling Side Kick helps your entire body:

The pelvic nerve root structures are optimally helped. The fact that the pelvic floor is challenged to help with balance and the hips have to gain full range, allows the nerves to slide in a wonderful long rotational motion as the leg moves. The range gained during this motion by the hip that is moving is full dynamic range – a range that is essential to a wondrous sexual experience!

Kneeling Side Kick

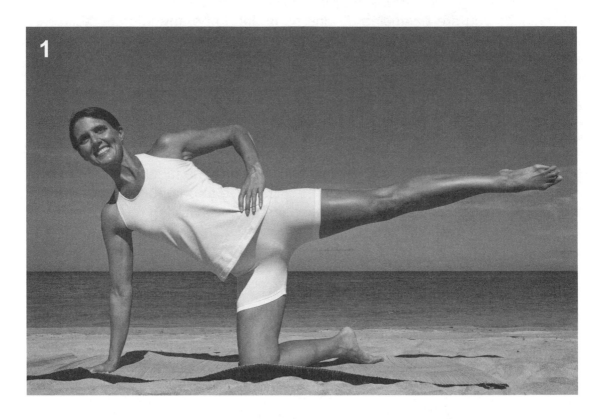

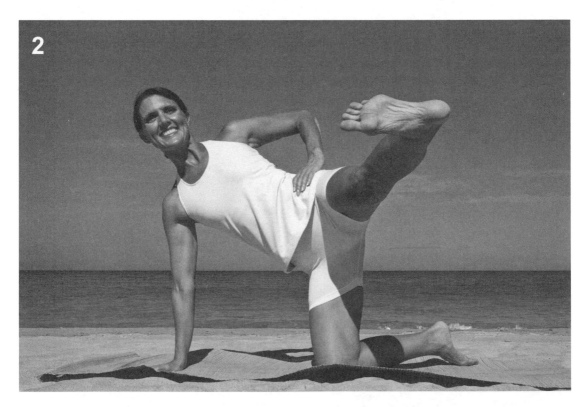

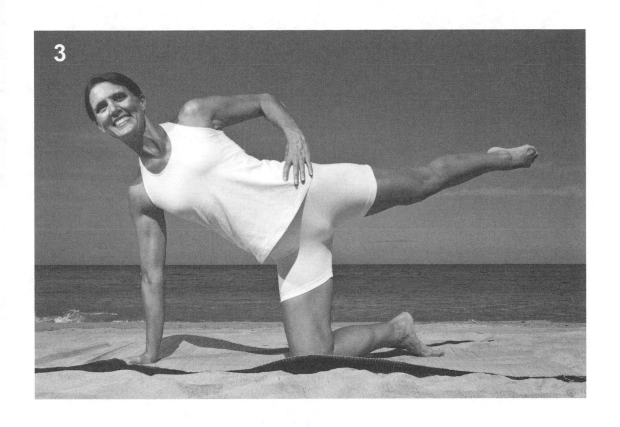

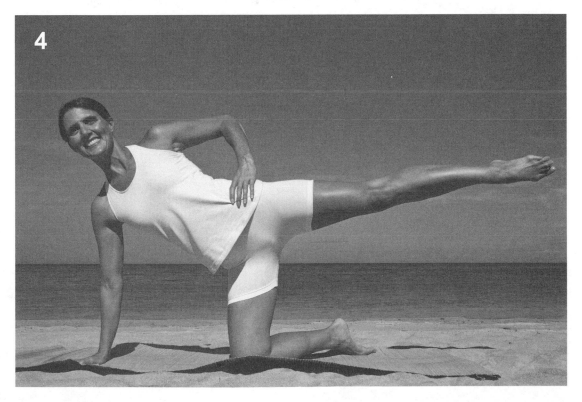

CHAPTER
FIVE

Pilates, Sex & The Aphrodisiac Diet

I want to take a moment and talk about diet and not just eating right but an aphrodisiac diet. Eating a well-balanced diet and adding aphrodisiac foods and herbs to your diet will not just boost your libido but boost your metabolism, energy level and control weight. Some of our most common foods and some you may enjoy daily are aphrodisiacs. What exactly is an aphrodisiac? An aphrodisiac is a substance that increases sexual desire. The name comes from Aphrodite, the Greek goddess of sexuality and love.

When you eat right your body feels, looks and functions better. Always remember to eat a balanced diet and incorporate these fun foods into your program to help boost your libido. Remember, everything in moderation especially some of the following decadent foods and try not to eat 1-2 hours before your Pilates program. This will help you find your center better and hollow out your abdominals. If the stomach is full it can be hard to "suck in your tummy." If you need to eat, have something light like a piece of fruit, veggies, piece of cheese or a choice from the following list of Aphrodisiac foods. Following is a list of some simple scrumptious additions you can add to your diet to boost your nervous system, help you build muscle and boost your sex drive!

Note:

These are only suggested foods and herbs to add to your diet. Please consult your doctor before you start any new diet program. This includes foods and herbs you are not familiar with or which are not part of your current diet, health and fitness program. Remember, everything in moderation. Bon Appétit!

Asparagus

The vitamin E in this green vegetable helps your body churn out hormones like testosterone, estrogen, and progesterone. These hormones circulate in your bloodstream and stimulate sexual responses like vaginal lubrication and increased blood flow to create sexual response. Three courses of asparagus were served to 19th century bridegrooms due to its reputed aphrodisiac powers. It is said that people who eat a lot of asparagus have many lovers.

Avocado

With all the Vitamin E in this amazing fruit your hormones like testosterone, estrogen and progesterone will be super charged. All these hormones circulate in your body getting you ready for super sex.

Bananas

Another reason to think about sex when you wrap your lips around this lush super fruit is bananas deliver potassium, a nutrient key to muscle strength. Potassium helps when you orgasm, causing the contractions to be super intense.

Celery

Celery is a stimulant and when the fresh root is eaten it strengthens the sex organs. Celery root contains an essential oil and the minerals iron, calcium, magnesium and sulphur.

Chilies

Capsaicin, a chemical found in fiery peppers, increases circulation to get blood pumping and stimulates nerve endings so you'll feel more turned on.

Chocolate

Cacao, the bean which chocolate is made from, contains the chemical phenylethylamine, a stimulant that conjures just the sort of subtle feelings of well being and excitement that make sex seem like a great idea.

Figs

In ancient Greece, new seasonal crops were celebrated with a frenzied copulation ritual.

Oysters

Oysters as an aphrodisiac sounds so cliché, but they really can spark friskiness. These shellfish contain a high level of zinc, a mineral that cranks up the production of testosterone, which has been linked to a higher sex drive.

Pomegranates

The pomegranate owes its passion power to antioxidants. Anti-oxidants protect the lining of blood vessels, allowing more blood to course through them. The bonus for you is increased genital sensitivity.

Red Wine

Besides relaxing you faster than a neck rub can, red wine contains reservatrol, an antioxidant that helps boost blood flow and improves circulation before and during intercourse.

Salmon

This hearty beautiful fish is packed with omega-3 fatty acids. Omega-3 fatty acids help keep sex-hormone production at its peak.

Vanilla

Ah, the beautiful and aromatic sweet vanilla bean. This magical bean mildly stimulates nerves, making sexual sensations feel even better.

Walnuts

Walnuts, like salmon, are also packed with omega-3 fatty acids, which keep hormone production up.

Watermelon

The juicy fruit of the watermelon contains the phytonutrient citrulline, which leads to an uptake in the amount of nitric oxide in your body. That spike in nitric oxide causes blood vessels to relax and speeds up blood circulation. As a result, you'll get more aroused in less time.

Herbs:

American Ginseng (origin: N. America)

American ginseng is used as general tonic that strengthens the body. It can be eaten fresh, or as a dried root infusion. The root was used by American Indians as a protective amulet and a love charm.

Basil (origin: South Asia, Europe)

Some varieties of Basil are used as spices, some for medical uses. Eat one leaf a day to express religious respect, maintain health, prosperity and fertility. The popular herb contains aphrodisiac powers and never gives you a boring sex life.

Cacao tree (origin: Central America)

Cacao is a mild stimulant whose ground beans can be made into a drink or chocolate. An ancient Indian recipe of cacao roasted beans are ground and dissolved in water, along with vanilla, cayenne pepper, matico pepper, pimento, and canella, and can be salted or sweetened with honey. Cacao was considered the "food of gods." Aztec prostitutes were paid in cacao. Cacao beans contain theobromine and caffeine, and the aphrodisiac phenylethylamine.

Cardamom (origin: Southeast Asia)

Stimulant, especially if added to coffee. The essential oil has an erotic effect on the body.

Cayenne Pepper (origin: Middle and South America)

Cayenne pepper is a stimulant when the fruit is fresh or dried. It is a hot food and enhances the sexual drive. Contains acrid substance capsaicin and tons of vitamin C. As with any herb or food avoid over usage.

Cola nut (origin: Central Africa)

In Central America cola nut can be chewed raw or the extract of the nut ingested. Ingesting cola nut is a stimulant used in love magic and was once used as currency in W Africa. Cola nut contains high concentrations of caffeine, theobromine and tannin.

Gotu Kola (origin: Asia)

Invigorating tonic which can be drunk as a tea or the plant can be eaten. Daily use of leaves or tea from dry leaves prolongs life and fires the sexuality. Leaves and seeds have alkaloid (vitamin X) that stimulates adrenal glands.

Garlic (origin: Southwestern Asia)

Garlic is a tonic and rejuvenates the body. When used as a spice garlic has a magic element to banish bad influences or vampires. Essential oils have an antibiotic and cell-activating effect. Garlic has been used as an aphrodisiac since the Egyptians. The Romans consecrated it to Ceres, the goddess of fertility.

Ginger (origin: South Asia)

The root of the ginger can be eaten or made into a tea. Ginger has properties of creating heat and brings fire into the body.

Gingko (origin: China, Japan)

The plant is a last surviving representative from the Mesozoic period, 240 million years ago. Grilled seeds are a very good aphrodisiac for men. In addition Ginkgo brings power to the lower abdomen.

Horseradish (origin: Southeast Europe)

When the root is eaten it has stimulating properties in the body. In fact the root often looks exactly like an erect penis. Like other pungent spices it promotes love. It's popular for renewing strength after sexual exhaustion. The root is rich in vitamin C, potassium, Calcium and magnesium, Iron and enzymes. Horseradish stimulates activity of the stomach and intestines and has expectorant, diuretic and warming effect on the body.

Licorice (origin: Europe, Asia)

Licorice is a great tonic when ingested as a tea or in powder form. Licorice is especially popular as an aphrodisiac among women.

Morning Glory (origin: America)

Morning glory seeds were considered the home of God and used in pre Columbian times for gynecological problems, divinatory and religious purposes. 2-4 seeds have direct affect on sexual drive. Morning glory seeds contain lysergic acid derivatives that cause uterine contractions.

Mustard (origin: Europe)

The ground seeds and plant of mustard promote virility; therefore monks were forbidden to eat mustard.

Rosemary (origin: Eurasia, N. Africa)

Rosemary has a strong erotic effect upon the skin and can be ingested as spice and can be added to a bath or to wine.

Saffron (origin: Asia, N. Africa)

Saffron has hot and dry qualities. It can be a stimulant or inebriant depending on dosage. Sun dried filaments that are ingested can strengthen the uterus and help treat menstrual problems and stimulates sexual desires for women. Essential oil evokes long, distinctive orgasms.

Wild Rose (Original origin unknown. Roses possibly inhabited the earth before humans.)

Wild Rose is an erotic stimulant, especially for women. Rose promotes love and magic. Rose petals can be used in tea or love potions and rose oil is often used as a perfume.

Ylang-Ylang (origin: Southwest Asia)

Ylang-Ylang increases eroticism and is prescribed to treat impotency and frigidity. The oil contains a variety of essential components and acids and can be used internally or externally. When Ylang-Ylang is mixed with coconut oil it creates a highly erotic body lotion. Yum!

History is rife with the human pursuit of aphrodisiacs in many forms. Scientific tests have proven that some aromas can cause a greater effect on the body than the actual ingestion of foods.

Many of the foods and herbs we have mentioned come in the form of essential oils, are used in perfumes or in cooking. Natural foodstuffs, herbs and spices act as a pheromone to communicate emotions by smell.

Sometimes I will place a couple of drops of my favorite essential oil on my Pilates mat to have the stimulating scent throughout my practice. Try some rose oil, rosemary or basil oil on your mat. It will motivate you and stimulate your Pilates practice and your love life.

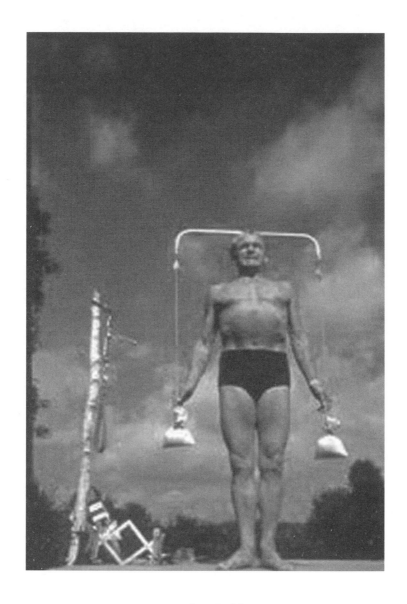

Joseph Pilates
"A lifetime of Health and Vitality!"

Conclusion

As you have progressed through the weeks of your Pilates for Sexual Enhancement program you may have noticed more than just a longer, stronger, more flexible body and enhanced sex life. Hopefully you feel a greater sense of balance both physically and mentally. Pilates like any fitness program is a way of life, meaning it is something that you carry with you all the time in the way you move, breath, approach life and treat yourself and others. Pilates is a program that can promote calmness, control, confidence and personal power both mentally and physically. We hope that your daily practice has given you a greater sense of yourself, your commitment to yourself, your health and given you an overall feeling of wellbeing. Of course our main goal with this program is to show you a Pilates program that not only enhances your life but your sex life as well.

Congratulations on your dedication and commitment to your mind and body. Maintain your commitment with daily practice and challenge yourself daily by doing 2 or 3 programs during the same practice.

Remember your commitment to yourself will project into your personal everyday life on every level.

Thank you for following our program we hope it made your life and your sex life that much more fabulous!

Glossary

Alcock's Tunnel - Ishiorectal fossa is a depression in the inferior pelvic bone and the "roof of this is formed by fascia, together these form the Alcock's tunnel and the pudendal nerve passes through this tunnel.

Antagonist muscle - Muscle that initiates the contraction.

Angonist - Muscle that works in opposition to the antagonist.

Atrophy - The partial or complete wasting away of a part of the body. Causes of atrophy can be poor nourishment, poor circulation, loss of hormonal support, loss of nerve supply to the target organ, disuse or lack of exercise or disease intrinsic to the tissue itself.

Concentric contraction - Contraction of a muscle where the muscle fibres shorten. An example of a concentric contraction is the raising of a weight during a bicep curl.

Diaphragm - Large muscle below the lungs, for abdominal strength and breathing.

Eccentric Contraction - Contraction of a muscle where the muscle fibres actively lengthen. Examples of this are walking, when the quadriceps (knee extensors) are active just after heel strike, while the knee flexes, or setting an object down gently (the arm flexors must be active to control the fall of the object). With increasing load on the muscle, a point is reached where, even though the muscle may be fully activated, it is forced to lengthen due to the high external load.

Erectile dysfunction - Lack of ability to gain a normal erection or maintain an erection.

Gynecology - Specialization in the medical field focused on women's health.

Ilipsoas muscle - A hip flexing muscles running from the front of the spine to the front of the hip.

Innervation - The nerve supply of the muscles, bones and organs

Ischium - Bones in the lower portion of the pelvis.

Libido - Sexual urge or desire.

Ligamentous Structures - Non-elastic fibrous connective tissue bands that provide structural support during movement of joints in the body.

Lumbar spine - Last 5 vertebrae in the spinal column.

Muscle fibres - Muscles are compiled by millions of small fibres

Nerve Roots - Where the central nervous system produces spinal nerves, exiting the spinal cord at each vertebral segment.

Nervous System - Complex system of nerves running throughout the entire body.

Nerve, Femoral - Large nerve running down the front of the thigh.

Nerve, Obturator - Nerve with transects the hip region deep in the muscles.

Nerve, Pudendal - Important nerves supplying and found in the pelvic floor, its responsible for proper functioning and control of urination, defecation and orgasm in both males and females. Located deep within the pelvic region, the pudendal nerve emerges from the base of the spinal cord (sacral area), and separates into three branches. One branch goes to the anal-rectal area. The second branch goes to the perineum - the sensitive area between the anus and penis or vagina. The third branch goes to the penis or clitoris itself.

Nerve, Peroneal - Nerve running along the outer side of the lower leg.

Nerve, Sciatic - Nerve which is found behind the hip and between the hamstrings, it is a large sensory and motor nerve running through the posterior hip and down between the hamstrings , branching in the leg to supply the lower extremity.

Nerve, Tibial - Nerve which is found behind the knee and runs down to the foot.

Neurodynamic - Relating the dynamic slide, glide and tensioning of the nerves as we move our body.

Neuralgia - Pain which originates from nerve dysfunction or injury.

Oscillation – Slow forward and back ward motion while performing a range of motion exercise.

Osseus - Bone structures.

Pelvis - The ring of bones at the base of the spinal column.

Piriformes - Large hip muscle controlling rotation in the hip.

Pubic Symphysis - Anterior joint in the pelvic ring.

Sacroiliac joint - Two large joints at the back of the pelvis.

Synergistic - May be defined as two or more things functioning together to produce a result not independently obtainable. The term synergy comes from the Greek word syn-ergos, meaning "working together."

Terminal Nerve Ending - Where the end of a nerve is found in a muscle.

Transverse Abdominus - Deepest stomach muscle for core strength.

Urology - Medical field specializing in the urinary system.

Urogenital diaphragm - The muscles that form the pelvic floor muscles.

Urogenic - Pain originating from the pelvic floor muscles or sexual organs.

References

1. Butler DS (1991), Mobilisation of the Nervous system, Churchill Livingstone, Melbourne, Australia.

2. Butler DS (2000), The Sensitive Nervous System, Noigroup Publications, Adelaide, Australia.

3. Franklin Eric N. (2002), Pelvic Power for Men and Women, Princeton Book Company, Hightstown, NJ, USA.

4. Massey P. (2009), The Anatomy of Pilates, North Atlantic Books, Berkley, CA, USA.

5. Kendall F. P., McCreary E.K., Provance P.G. (2005), Muscles, Testing and Functions, Lippincott Williams & Wilkins, Baltimore, MD, USA.

6. Butler, D.S. (2005), The Neurodynamic Techniques, Noigroup Publications, Adelaide, Australia.

7. Calais-Germain, B. (1993), Anatomy of Movement, Eastland Press Inc., Seattle, WA, USA.

8. Siler, B. (2006), Your Ultimate Pilates Body Challenge, Broadway books, New York, NY, USA.

9. Bø K., Berghmans B., Mørkved S., Van Kampen M., (2007) Evidence-Based Physical Therapy for the Pelvic Floor, Churchill Livingstone Elsevier,Edinburgh, UK.

10. Calais-Germain, B. (2003), The Female Pelvis – Anatomy and Exercises, Eastland Press Inc., Seattle, WA, USA.

11. Gilman S. MD, Winans Newman S. Ph.D. (1996), Essentials of Clinical Neuroanatomy and Neurophysiology, F.A. Davis Company, Philadelphia, PA, USA

12. Wolf-Heidegger, (2004) The Color Atlas of Human Anatomy, Sterling Publishing Co, New York, NY, USA

13. Menezes, A, (1999), The Complete Guide to the Pilates Method: From Lower Back Pain to Muscle Conditioning, Pilates Institute of Australasia, North Sydney, NSW, Australia.

Index

Notes

Notes

Notes